PEDIGREE ANALYSIS IN HUMAN GENETICS

The Johns Hopkins Series in Contemporary Medicine and Public Health

Also of interest in this series:

Analysis of Human Genetic Linkage
Jurg Ott

Pedigree Analysis in Human Genetics

ELIZABETH A. THOMPSON

DEPARTMENT OF PURE MATHEMATICS
AND MATHEMATICAL STATISTICS,
UNIVERSITY OF CAMBRIDGE

The Johns Hopkins University Press
BALTIMORE AND LONDON

©1986 The Johns Hopkins University Press
All rights reserved
Printed in the United States of America

The Johns Hopkins University Press
701 West 40th Street
Baltimore, Maryland 21211
The Johns Hopkins Press Ltd, London

*The paper in this book is acid-free and meets
the guidelines for permanence and durability of
the Committee on Production Guidelines for Book
Longevity of the Council on Library Resources.*

LIBRARY OF CONGRESS CATALOGING IN PUBLICATION DATA
Thompson, E. A. (Elizabeth Alison), 1949–
   Pedigree analysis in human genetics.
   (The Johns Hopkins series in contemporary medicine
and public health)
   Bibliography: p.
   Includes index.
   1. Human genetics—Statistical methods.   2. Human population
genetics—Statistical methods.   3. Medical genetics—Statistical methods.
I. Title.   II. Series. [DNLM: 1. Genetics, Medical.   2. Models,
Genetic.   3. Pedigree.   4. Probability.   QH 431 T469p]
QH431.T47   1985   573.2′1   85-9821
ISBN 0-8018-2790-6 (alk. paper)

Contents

Appendixes

List of Figures

List of Tables

Preface

The scope of pedigree analysis is wider than many of its students and practitioners recognize. In the United States the subject is usually associated with genetic epidemiology; on the continent of Europe it is more often taken to relate to inferences concerning the genealogical structure itself—at the most basic level, paternity testing. In fact, genetic data on a set of interrelated individuals may be viewed from either of these perspectives, or from others. Questions of the genetic determinants for medical familial traits, the reconstruction of genealogies from genetic data, the extinction of genes in small populations, the ancestry of certain alleles or predictions of their future distributions and effects, all involve the analysis of data on large and complex genealogies. Although each genealogy and data set provides its own particular structure and questions of interest, an approach to solving one question can provide insights into others.

A main theme of this text is that problems involving large genealogies have much in common. The single problem of computing probabilities of observed genetic data on a given pedigree structure is the basis of the solution to each. It is the wealth of different ways in which these probabilities can be viewed that provides continuing variety to the subject.

The present text grew out of a series of eight lectures given to graduate students in statistics in 1981 and again in 1982. The aim of the lectures was not to challenge the students' statistical and mathematical abilities; rather, it was to provide a broad introduction to the variety of pedigree analysis topics, thereby motivating some students to delve more deeply into the many intriguing applied problems. The objective of this book is the same. So, too, are the theoretical ideas, but the mathematical formalism of the lectures has been considerably reduced, making the text accessible to those with little mathematical training. Where theory is required in order to provide an understanding of results, it is presented through detailed discussion of a particular example rather than through intimidating theoretical formulations. Each chapter is based on one lecture of the original series, and is designed to cover one topic, broadly independent of the others, although the same ideas follow through.

Apart from the first two chapters, which introduce the basic groundwork, each chapter is motivated by a study of a particular data set. This is done not only to make the material more accessible but also to express my belief that the applied problems should determine the theoretical presentation. In studies of South American Indians (chapter 3) the reconstruction of genealogies from genetic data is a relevant problem, while questions of gene identity and gene extinction are of practical importance in analyzing the ancestry of alleles in a complex Mennonite-Amish genealogy (chapter 4). The small number of founders of the Tristan da Cunhan population suggests the real possibility of tracing the ancestral origins of current polymorphic genes (chapter 5). Problems of genetic modeling and counseling are considered, but mainly in the context of Mendelian traits segregating in the large genealogies of small isolated populations; studies of a dermatoglyphic trait in a Habbanite isolate (chapter 6) and of lymphoreticular malignancies in western Newfoundland (chapter 7) are presented. In the final chapter some questions of sampling and ascertainment are discussed. Sampling in pedigree analysis is a complicated problem, but it is also an important one. The basic ideas can and should be presented to current and future practitioners in the area.

Since I have chosen to present pedigree analysis through studies in which I have been involved, there are limitations and biases in the resulting text. One such bias is the manner in which references are cited. Rather than spread references throughout the text, I have included a section on further reading at the end of each chapter. The references in these sections are restricted to basic texts, major relevant theoretical papers, and papers relating to the data analyzed in each chapter. These sources will not only enable readers to pursue any given topic more deeply but will also lead them to related studies and references that it has not been possible to include here.

A second limitation is the type of genetic traits considered. Although a chapter is included on some of the more complex genetic models now employed in genetic epidemiology, primary emphasis is placed on more simply determined traits. Mendelian traits provide ample scope for analysis, and they are the type of data with which I have worked. Complex genetic models present complications when discussed in conjunction with large and complex genealogies. However, the omission of such models from the text is not intended as a denial of their relevance in the analysis of complex traits.

Another area of genetics which receives little attention in the present text is linkage analysis. With the rapid growth in the number of established DNA polymorphisms and the resulting possibilities for mapping the human genome, linkage analysis has already altered the field of genetic epidemiology and will undoubtedly play a part in studies of genetic isolates and large genealogies. For this reason I have included linkage analyses in chapters 6 and 7. However, these two applications are surely crude preliminaries to the future of this particular area of study.

A final conscious limitation is the restriction of examples to human genealogies. This again reflects my own biases, but it also results in a more coherent text. Examples from diverse species might obscure the unifying feature of such studies—a probability on a pedigree that can be viewed in diverse ways. However, problems of genealogical reconstruction, genetic determinants of traits, gene extinction, and allelic origins also arise in other species, which have their own genetic isolates and extended pedigrees (known or unknown). It is hoped that the present text will be of interest to zoologists and population ecologists as well as to all those who study human populations.

I am grateful to many people for helping me complete this text. First, to all those with whom I have collaborated on applications of the methodology and whose data prompted new questions and required new approaches. Some of these are acknowledged in the relevant chapters, but there are others to whom I am no less grateful. Second, more specific thanks are due to Pat Stewart. All the diagrams of genealogies in standard classical form were done using her version of the Landre-Salmon pedigree-drawing program on the Cambridge University IBM computer. I am grateful for her help and patience with my many requests for minor alterations in options and formats. Third, my thanks are due to all those who read and commented upon any part of the text. In particular, I would like to express my debt to Tom Meagher, who read and reread almost all of the text and whose encouragement was instrumental in ensuring its completion. Last but not least, I am grateful to the students who attended the lectures. Their questions and criticisms forced me to examine foundations more carefully and to clarify my assumptions. In particular, I would like to thank Patty Solomon, Alun Thomas, and Daniel Goodman.

PEDIGREE ANALYSIS IN HUMAN GENETICS

1. A Brief Introduction to Human Genetics

1.1. Genes, segregation, and diploidy

Most of the content of this chapter may be familiar, but it is convenient to summarize the fundamental genetic facts on which the remainder of the text is built and to introduce some basic terminology. No other specific genetic knowledge will be assumed, but those whose training is in other areas may find it useful to consult additional texts (for example, those cited at the end of the chapter) to gain a more general overview of the genetic background. Likewise, the required probability and statistical theory is covered in the appendixes. Although these should suffice for a first reading of the text, and will provide a convenient summary of the relevant ideas, those who wish to pursue the subject more deeply will need some knowledge of elementary probability and statistics.

Mendel postulated his First Law in 1866, on the basis of studies of pea plants. He postulated that discrete entities, which he called *characters* but which are now called *genes*, pass from parents to offspring. Rewording his postulates in modern terminology, he suggested that each plant carries two genes that determine any given characteristic. That is, two genes determine whether the flowers of the pea plant are red, pink, or white. Two other genes determine whether the pea pod is rough or smooth, and so on. Further, one of the two genes is received from the male parent plant, the other from the female parent plant, and in the formation of offspring a random one of the two genes is passed (that is, *segregates*) to the offspring. Different offspring of the same parent result from *independent* segregations. This scenario is shown in figure 1, where the genes determining a given trait of interest are labeled $g_1, \ldots, g_6$. Four types of offspring can result from the mating shown; each does so with probability 1/4. Knowledge of the genes segregating on one occasion conveys no information about the next. Figure 1 also introduces some standard notation. Males are denoted by squares and females by circles; in this text a triangle denotes an individual of either sex. A pair of parents is connected by a horizontal line, and a vertical line descends to the offspring. Where there is more than one child of the same parent pair, these are shown under a second horizontal sibship line.

Although elegantly simple, Mendel's First Law covers much of genetics. The consequences are far-reaching and lead to complicated distributions of traits in populations. In several respects Mendel was lucky; the first being that peas, like humans, are *diploid*. That is, they do indeed carry genes in pairs, which can therefore segregate in the way described. Simple

Figure 1. Segregation of genes under Mendel's First Law.
□ = male; ○ = female; △ = either sex.

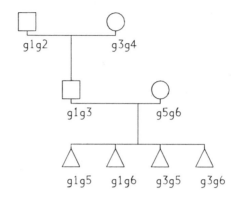

organisms, such as amoebae, carry only one gene for each trait, and have only one parent. Some plants carry four, and segregation is then a more complicated procedure. Other numbers also are possible.

1.2. Alleles, genotypes, and loci

The genes carried by individuals may be labeled according to *type*, depending on their effects on observed traits. The alternative types affecting the same characteristic are known as *alleles*. For example, there might be two types of gene affecting flower color, one tending to produce red flowers and the other white. These could be labeled as the R and W alleles. Every individual has two genes controlling its color; it could have two R alleles (RR), two W alleles (WW), or one of each (RW). If it has one of each, it is irrelevant which comes from the mother and which from the father: $RW = WR$. The unordered pair of alleles carried by an individual is its *genotype*; the three possible genotypes here are RR, RW, and WW. Generally, alleles will be denoted a_i, $i = 1, \ldots, s$, when there are s possible alleles. The genotypes are then $a_i a_j$ ($i \leq j$). That is, an individual with one a_3 allele and one a_1 allele is conventionally given genotype $a_1 a_3$ (not $a_3 a_1$). Individuals with two copies of one allele ($i = j$) are *homozygotes*. If the two alleles are different, the individual is a *heterozygote*. A homozygous parent must pass on to each child a gene of the only allelic type he carries, while a heterozygote passes on either one of his two alleles, each with probability 1/2. Thus, Mendelian segregation gives the genotype probabilities of a child, given the genotypes of his parents. The probabilities for a two-allele (*diallelic*) locus are shown in table 1.

The pair of genes controlling a given trait are called genes at a single *locus*. For example, there is a locus for pea flower color, a locus for pod

Table 1. Offspring genotype probabilities under Mendelian segregation at a diallelic locus

| | Offspring genotype | | | | |
| | Autosomal or female X-linked | | | Male X-linked | |
Parent genotypes	a_1a_1	a_1a_2	a_2a_2	a_1	a_2
a_1a_1, a_1a_1	1	0	0	—	—
a_1a_1, a_1a_2 (*)	$\frac{1}{2}$	$\frac{1}{2}$	0	—	—
a_1a_1, a_2a_2 (*)	0	1	0	—	—
a_1a_2, a_1a_2	$\frac{1}{4}$	$\frac{1}{2}$	$\frac{1}{4}$	—	—
a_1a_2, a_2a_2 (*)	0	$\frac{1}{2}$	$\frac{1}{2}$	—	—
a_2a_2, a_2a_2	0	0	1	—	—
a_1a_1, a_1	1	0	0	1	0
a_1a_2, a_1	$\frac{1}{2}$	$\frac{1}{2}$	0	$\frac{1}{2}$	$\frac{1}{2}$
a_2a_2, a_1	0	1	0	0	1
a_1a_1, a_2	0	1	0	1	0
a_1a_2, a_2	0	$\frac{1}{2}$	$\frac{1}{2}$	$\frac{1}{2}$	$\frac{1}{2}$
a_2a_2, a_2	0	0	1	0	1

Note: (*) = or vice versa.

texture, and so on. A locus may also be thought of as a position in the *genome*, that is, the long sequence of DNA bases that are in fact the genetic material. These chemical bases code for certain amino acids that together form the actual protein and enzyme constituents of an individual. For example, a certain part might be termed the "flower color locus," since it codes for the genes determining flower color. Fortunately, the traits considered by Mendel are *single-locus* traits. More complex traits may be affected by the types of genes found at several different loci.

Now, the DNA in a cell is divided into chromosomes—substrings of the genetic material. In the formation of new cells, or of *gametes* (sperm or ova), it is the chromosomes that segregate, rather than individual genes. Every normal cell of every human individual contains 46 chromosomes. Of these, 44 are the *autosomes*, consisting of 22 pairs. One of each pair was received from the mother, the other from the father. An *autosomal locus* is situated at some position on one of these 22 autosomes. The maternal gene is the gene on the chromosome received from the mother; the paternal gene is the gene in the same position on the chromosome received from the father. The remaining two chromosomes are sex chromosomes. For a human female, these are effectively a further pair of autosomes, known as X chromosomes, one being received from the mother, the other from the father. She will pass a copy of a randomly chosen one of the two to each of her

Figure 2. Sex determination and the segregation of X chromosomes

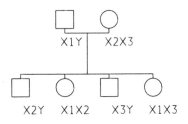

children. However, a male has only one X chromosome, received from his mother. His 46th chromosome is a small Y chromosome, which is a copy of the Y chromosome in his father. Figure 2 shows the segregation of sex chromosomes.

1.3. Phenotypes and the determination of traits

The observable character of an individual with respect to some trait of interest is his *phenotype* for that trait. A fundamental step in specifying the genetic basis of a trait is to define the relationship between genotype and phenotype. This relationship varies between traits, and for many traits is difficult to specify precisely. Again, Mendel was fortunate in that the traits he studied were mostly dichotomous traits determined by just two alleles, a_1 and a_2. There are, then, three genotypes. If $a_1 a_2$ individuals are phenotypically indistinguishable from $a_1 a_1$ individuals, the a_1 allele is said to be *dominant* (to a_2), the a_2 *recessive* (to a_1). If all three genotypes are distinguishable, the alleles are *codominant*. If all individuals having a certain character must carry an a_1 allele, a_1 is said to be the allele *for* the trait. If this allele is dominant, all $a_1 a_1$ and $a_1 a_2$ individuals will have the character, and the trait will also be said to be dominant. Conversely, if a_1 is the recessive allele, the trait will be limited to $a_1 a_1$ individuals and will then be described as a recessive trait. In this case, $a_1 a_2$ individuals are known as *carriers*, for, although phenotypically normal, they carry the allele for the trait. The child of two carriers has probability 1/4 of being of the $a_1 a_1$ genotype. Table 2 shows these standard genotype-phenotype relationships. Similar terminology applies to X-linked characteristics, which are determined by alleles at loci on the X chromosome. Here, males have only one gene affecting the trait, and dominance or recessivity does not apply, while a female may be phenotypically normal but carry one copy of an allele for a recessive X-linked trait. Since a male receives his only X chromosome from his mother, each of a carrier female's sons has probability 1/2 of being affected (see table 1). None of the studies in this text relates to X-linked traits, and therefore the theory will be developed entirely in the context of

Table 2. Phenotypes of individuals for traits determined by a simple relationship between phenotype and genotype at a single locus

Genotype	Dominant trait (a_1 dominant to a_2)	Recessive trait (a_1 recessive to a_2)	General dichotomous trait: Probabilities of characteristic T
$a_1 a_1$	(affected) [rare/unknown]	affected	$p(T \mid a_1 a_1)$
$a_1 a_2$	affected	normal carrier	$p(T \mid a_1 a_2)$
$a_2 a_2$	normal	normal	$p(T \mid a_2 a_2)$
a_1	affected	affected	$p(T \mid a_1)$
a_2	normal	normal	$p(T \mid a_2)$

autosomal loci. Although a parallel development for X-linked loci is possible, it will not be pursued.

The above description covers the simplest possible genotype-phenotype relationships. In fact, genotype may not determine phenotype precisely; the characteristics of an individual may depend on age, sex, environment, or even on other genetic loci. There will then be a genotype-dependent set of probabilities for the character (table 2). Another category is loci with multiple alleles. These include the blood-group and enzyme loci, where there can be many gene products. One good example is the ABO blood-group system. There are three alleles, *A*, *B*, and *O*, and hence six genotypes. However, there are only four phenotypes, as only *A* and *B* are codominant. Both these alleles are dominant to *O*. Thus, the *AA* and *AO* genotypes are phenotypically indistinguishable; both give blood type A. Similarly, *BB* and *BO* both give blood type B. The O blood group corresponds only to the recessive *OO* genotype, while *AB* individuals are also distinguishable from other genotypes. Clearly, with more alleles there are many alternative patterns of dominance between alleles. As a system is more closely investigated, more alleles are discovered, and more come to be regarded as codominant due to the increasing numbers of tests to separate the genotypes phenotypically. For the ultimate data on DNA sequence, all "alleles" are codominant and the number that are theoretically possible is greater than the number of *Homo sapiens* that have existed.

1.4. Population frequencies of alleles and genotypes

Different alleles occur in different populations with different frequencies. The *B* allele of the ABO system has frequency 7 percent in Europe, 15 percent in Africa, and 30 percent in parts of Asia, but is absent from Amerindians. In large populations, frequencies remain fairly stable over the generations, but in small populations chance segregations can cause marked fluctuations. A fundamental idea in population genetics is that of a *population allele frequency* (often called a *gene frequency*), this being interpreted as the probability that a randomly chosen gene from the population will be of a given allelic type.

Suppose that at a given autosomal locus there are s alleles, $a_1, \ldots, a_s$, and that the allele frequencies are $p_1, \ldots, p_s$ ($\Sigma_1^s p_i = 1$). Now, an individual has two genes. If his genes can be regarded as independently chosen from a very large (in fact, infinite) gene pool with the above frequencies, then

$$\left. \begin{array}{l} \text{the probability that both his genes are of type } a_i \text{ is } p_i^2; \\ \text{the probability that he has genotype } a_i a_j \ (i < j) \text{ is } 2p_i p_j; \end{array} \right\} \tag{1}$$

recall that the genotype is the unordered pair, so the a_i allele may be chosen and then the a_j allele, or vice versa, giving the factor of 2. In a very large population in which individuals mate completely at random, these will be the genotype frequencies after one generation of mating, and will so remain over successive generations. These frequencies are known as the *Hardy-Weinberg* equilibrium frequencies. They provide a useful basis for assigning probabilities to genotypes, although most populations will, for a variety of demographic and genetic reasons, show deviations from these genotype proportions. In fact, in finite populations, the allele frequencies themselves cannot be expected to remain unchanged.

Pursuing further this idea of a hypothetical infinite pool of alleles from which individuals can be constructed, suppose that there are two possibilities for each individual. Suppose that with probability f an individual has two genes that are copies of the same gene in the underlying pool, in which case he must be a homozygote and will have genotype $a_i a_i$ with probability p_i. For the remaining probability $(1 - f)$, let us assume that his two genes will be independently chosen as before. Then, overall, the genotype probabilities will be as follows:

$$\left. \begin{array}{ll} \text{for genotype } a_i a_i & f p_i + (1 - f) p_i^2 = p_i^2 + f p_i (1 - p_i); \\ \text{for genotype } a_i a_j \ (i < j) & (1 - f) \, 2 p_i p_j. \end{array} \right\} \tag{2}$$

Besides providing genotype probabilities, under this particular abstract sampling model, which will in fact turn out to have practical application, the introduction of the additional parameter f allows for more scope in the specification of genotype probabilities. Under the model, f must lie between 0 and 1, and there will be a deficiency of heterozygotes compared to the Hardy-Weinberg frequencies. However, in general, f may be taken as any number that maintains positive frequencies (2), and thus can be used to express genotype probabilities in populations in which there is an excess of heterozygotes. This additional freedom, in which f is any parameter to be fitted, should not be confused with its derivation as a probability in sampling from an infinite gene pool.

Since the hypothetical infinite gene pool cannot exist, we are faced with fundamental problems concerning the precise definitions and meaning of allele frequencies. In small populations, these lead to practical problems as well. When all individuals are related, they carry copies of the same genes. Should copies be counted multiply, or only once? And how far should relationships be traced to discover which genes are copies of the same original? Ultimately, all copies of an allele may descend from only one original. The actual allele frequency *in* a population is easily comprehended but is not often useful. For future predictions, the frequency in the breeding generation is more relevant, but again that is not easily specified precisely. More often, in a genealogical study, it is necessary to give a probability for the genotypes of founders (original ancestors) of a genealogy. The genes in descendant individuals are then copies of the various founder genes, having descended by segregations with probabilities given by Mendel's First Law. Then the relevant frequency is that in an infinite gene pool, of which a gene in the founder individual may be taken as a random member. Such a gene pool is difficult to visualize. The founders of a genealogy may not be independent immigrants, but simply individuals to whom ancestry has been traced. The relevant gene pool will change if further tracing of a genealogy is undertaken. Before a study is undertaken, the genealogical relationships in a population may not be known. Even afterward, they may not be known with any certainty.

Although the basis for allele frequencies and for Hardy-Weinberg (or other) genotype probabilities may be hard to define or to justify, it seldom involves practical problems. The ability to assign a prior probability to a genotype is crucial, but the exact numerical value assigned seldom matters. Provided sensible assumptions are made, reliable inferences should result.

1.5. The forces of evolution

This text is not concerned with the evolutionary changes of allele frequencies that occur in all populations, yet it is important to recognize that such frequencies are a transient characteristic and have no absolute meaning. The three major directional forces that affect allele frequencies are mutation, selection, and migration. In addition, because all natural populations are finite each generation is only a particular realization of all the events that could have occurred in the segregation of genes from parents to offspring. Even if, on the average, the characteristics of offspring were those of their parents, over a period of time random fluctuations would occur. If the same genealogical process occurred again (the same individuals producing the same offspring), one would not expect to see the same alleles present in descendant individuals. In the small populations of interest in pedigree analysis, this process of random genetic drift can have major effects, which are central to the nature of data observations. However, it will not be necessary to consider the formal analysis of this population process, for it is simply a consequence of the operation of Mendelian segregation in genealogies, and the analysis of the latter is the basis of pedigree analysis.

The process of mutation involves the random change of the allelic type of a gene upon its segregation from parent to offspring. Although this change occurs only with very small probability, over many generations a gene will differ in type from its ancestral originator. However, although mutation is the ultimate source of genetic variability in populations, for the limited time span over which detailed human genealogies can be known it is a negligible force. It is rarely the explanation of an individual's possessing an allele not present in either of his putative parents, although it is always a possible one.

Selection is the differing viability and/or fertility of individuals, this variation being genotype dependent. This viability differential can have nonnegligible effects over the period of a genealogy. However, selection forces are seldom known with sufficient accuracy to be incorporated into analyses. They may be slight, and although important to the long-term genotypic profile of a population or species, irrelevant to the analysis of data on a genealogy. Alternatively, or additionally, they may be complex, depending on genotypes at several loci, and so not be sufficiently specific for inclusion. Extreme forms of selection, such as the nonviability of individuals affected by a trait under analysis, are of course relevant and should be included. More general forms of selection remain background factors that limit the generality of inferences based on specific genealogies rather than factors that affect the analysis of data on those genealogies.

Migration of individuals between and within populations is the third major force of population genetics, and can have substantial effects over short periods. Pedigree analysis is the analysis of data on specified individuals, so migration as a population force on population allele frequencies is not relevant. Data on the migration of individuals, or on the origins of immigrants to a genealogy or small population, however, may convey important genotypic information.

1.6. Chromosomes and linkage

Mendel stated as his Second Law that the genes controlling different traits are independently inherited. Again, this proposition depended on the precise traits he studied. Biologically, it is chromosomes that segregate, and genes at loci that are adjacent on a chromosome will not segregate independently. If, in a certain individual, g_1 and g_1^* are the paternal genes at loci L and L^*, and g_2 and g_2^* are the maternal genes, then that individual's offspring will tend to receive either g_1 and g_1^* or g_2 and g_2^*. This tendency is not absolute; it is possible for a *recombination* to occur between loci on the same chromosome. The offspring then receives g_1 and g_2^* or g_2 and g_1^*. The probabilities of the four events are shown in figure 3, parameterized by the linkage parameter, or *recombination fraction*, r. If the loci are very close on a chromosome, recombination is improbable and r is small. If they are on different chromosomes, or distant on the same one, $r = 1/2$ and Mendel's Second Law holds. One aim of pedigree analysis is the detection of linkage, for data on extended families can provide powerful evidence for (or against) it. Essentially, the aim is to estimate the extent to which the paternal gene at one locus does indeed segregate with the paternal gene at another (and likewise, of course, the maternal genes).

In many cases, offspring genotype probabilities are unchanged by linkage. For example, if (g_1, g_1^*) are of allelic types (a_1, a_1^*) and (g_2, g_2^*) are (a_2, a_1^*), then the chromosomes segregating to offspring are 50 percent $a_1 a_1^*$ and 50 percent $a_2 a_1^*$, regardless of whether or not recombination has occurred (see table 3). Only if the parent individual is heterozygous at both loci (a *double heterozygote*) is linkage effective, the offspring chromosomes then having the probabilities shown in table 3. Consider an infinite, random-mating population, and linkage between two autosomal loci, at

Figure 3. The segregation of chromosomes carrying linked loci. Note that for one parent all four genes are distinguished. Offspring may receive either g_1 or g_2 at the first locus and either g_1^* or g_2^* at the other, but the combination (g_1, g_1^*) has higher probability than the combination (g_1, g_2^*), since the former pairing is that in the parent while the latter requires a crossover, an event that occurs with the probability r independently for each offspring. Children whose gene combinations are the result of a recombination are known as recombinants; the others are known as nonrecombinants. Similar segregation events apply to the maternal gene of each offspring, but for simplicity she is assumed to carry two identical chromosomes, each carrying the genes g_3 and g_3^*, so each child carries the same combination, whether or not a crossover occurs between the two loci.

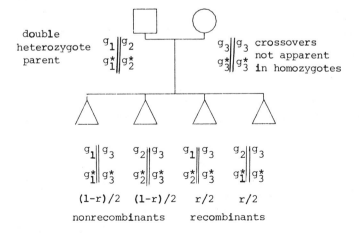

Table 3. Segregation probabilities for a parent genotype at two linked loci, with recombinations at rate r

Parent genotype $g_1 g_1^* / g_2 g_2^*$	Combination of alleles segregating to offspring			
	$a_1 a_1^*$	$a_1 a_2^*$	$a_2 a_1^*$	$a_2 a_2^*$
$a_1 a_1^* / a_2 a_1^*$	$1/2$	0	$1/2$	0
$a_1 a_1^* / a_2 a_2^*$	$1/2(1-r)$	$1/2 r$	$1/2 r$	$1/2(1-r)$
$a_1 a_2^* / a_2 a_1^*$	$1/2 r$	$1/2(1-r)$	$1/2(1-r)$	$1/2 r$

each of which there are two alleles. Let the frequencies of the chromosomes $a_1 a_1^*$, $a_1 a_2^*$, $a_2 a_1^*$, and $a_2 a_2^*$ be y_{11}, y_{12}, y_{21}, and y_{22}, and let

$$D_y = y_{11} y_{22} - y_{12} y_{21}. \tag{3}$$

Thus, D_y is a measure of the population association between alleles at the two loci. Consider the parentage of a current $a_1 a_1^*$ chromosome in the preceding generation, in which the chromosome frequencies were x_{11}, x_{12}, x_{21}, and x_{22}. Then

$$y_{11} = x_{11}(1 - x_{22}) \quad \text{(the other chromosome in the parental individual was not } a_2 a_2^*\text{)}$$
$$+ x_{11} x_{22}(1 - r) \quad \text{(the other parental chromosome was } a_2 a_2^*, \text{ but there was no recombination)}$$
$$+ x_{12} x_{21} r \quad \text{(the parental chromosome was } a_1 a_2^*, \text{ which recombined with } a_2 a_1^*\text{)}.$$

Or

$$y_{11} = x_{11} - r D_x,$$

and similarly

$$y_{22} = x_{22} - r D_x, \quad y_{12} = x_{12} + r D_x, \quad \text{and } y_{21} = x_{21} + r D_x,$$

so that

$$D_y = y_{11} y_{22} - y_{12} y_{21} = D_x - r D_x (x_{11} + x_{22} + x_{12} + x_{21})$$
$$+ r^2 D_x^2 - r^2 D_x^2$$
$$= D_x (1 - r), \tag{4}$$

and D is decreased by a factor $(1 - r)$ each generation.

Linkage is thus neither a necessary nor a sufficient condition for association of alleles at different loci within the individuals of a population. However, tight linkage (r is small) maintains associations caused by selection, mixing of populations, random fluctuations, and other population forces, whereas without linkage ($r = 1/2$) these associations decay rapidly

$(D_y = D_x / 2)$. Linkage can result in allelic associations within a single extended genealogy, since the chance combinations in ancestral individuals with many descendants will tend to be maintained in those descendants. Such associations may thus be indicative of linkage (see sections 6.5 and 7.5), but this can be tested only by analyzing the joint segregation pattern at the loci in question.

1.7. More complex aspects of genetics

So far this chapter has dealt only with qualitative traits. Many quantitative traits are partially genetically determined, but factors such as environment tend to play a greater role. A quantitative trait could in theory be determined by genotype, even by the genotype at a single autosomal locus. There need be no intrinsic difference between the determination of a quantitative trait and that of a qualitative one. For example, each genotype might provide a mean and variance for the distribution of height, with the actual height of an individual being distributed on either side of the relevant genotypic mean, the value being determined by the environmental history of the individual. Such a model is described in section 6.1, but could be realistic only if there were many alleles and there were then many unknown parameters (the mean and variances). A form of the model which is mathematically more tractable is to consider the limit of more and more independent loci, each contributing smaller and smaller amounts to a character. In the limit the "genotype" of an individual is a variable taking a numerical value; that is, a *polygenic component* that is itself quantitative. The probability distribution of the polygenic component for an offspring depends on the parental values; as such, it is a continuous analog of the Mendelian segregation probabilities of table 1. Polygenic models play an important role in genetic epidemiology, and will be described more fully in section 6.2, but the main focus of this text will be upon qualitative traits determined by single Mendelian loci.

Other aspects of human biology and geography complicate the analysis of genetic traits. One important one is nonrandom mating. That is, the genotype of an individual is not independent of that of his spouse, with resulting distortions in the genotype probabilities of offspring. The Hardy-Weinberg frequencies will no longer obtain, and one factor determining the parameter f in equation (2) can be such dependence between the types of maternal and paternal gametes. Nonrandom mating can result from demographic subdivision of a population, partial or total, by age or by geography, and may have important effects on variation within a population. Such effects on population characteristics are the basis of many population genetics analyses (see Cavalli-Sforza and Bodmer 1971, for example). Nonrandom mating can also result from an active assortment of individuals by phenotype. This will occur particularly for quantitative traits, such as height, and will not apply to most of the analyses of this text. Alternatively, or additionally, there may be preferences or prohibitions of marriages between individuals in certain genealogical relationships. The expected phenotypic effects of such behavior are the subject of theoretical analyses; some models are described by Jacquard (1974). In this text, data are analyzed under a specified (known or hypothesized) genealogy. The data are specific to individuals rather than being population characteristics. Any genealogically based mating pattern, and its genetic consequences on the characteristics of individuals, are thus subsumed within the analysis.

1.8. Joint and conditional probabilities

The formulas enabling probabilities of events to be transformed and manipulated will be found in appendix 1, but the ideas of joint and conditional probability are so central to the development of the theory and methodology of pedigree analysis that the definitions and notation are also introduced here. The probability of an event, that B has genotype $a_i a_i$, for example, will be denoted by $P(B$ is $a_i a_i)$. Probabilities are usually dependent on some implicit underlying assumptions, such as Mendelian segregation. Where alternatives to such assumptions are to be considered, it may be necessary to specify them explicitly, in which case they will be placed to the right of a vertical bar ($|$), read *given*; for example,

$$P(B \text{ is } a_i a_i \mid \text{Hardy-Weinberg equilibrium}) = p_i^2.$$

There are other assumptions here, both genetic (an autosomal locus) and notational (the allele frequency of a_i is p_i), but it would normally be only the Hardy-Weinberg assumption to which an alternative might be considered [such as the alternative of equation (2)].

In addition, it will often be necessary to consider events conditional upon others, as well as upon underlying model assumptions. For example, if a mother, M, has genotype $a_1 a_3$, her child, B, will be $a_2 a_3$ only if he receives the a_3 allele from her (probability 1/2) and an a_2 allele from his father. If this father is assumed to be a random member of the population, this gene is of type a_2 with probability p_2; thus,

$$P(B \text{ is } a_2 a_3 \mid M \text{ is } a_1 a_3) = (1/2)p_2. \tag{5}$$

Again, other assumptions are implicitly given in this probability (in particular, a random-mating assumption that will be employed in all the examples of this section), but the particular event for which one might wish to consider alternatives is the genotype of a putative mother. Of course, it is possible to condition upon several events; for example,

$$P(B \text{ is } a_2 a_3 \mid M \text{ is } a_1 a_3, F \text{ is } a_1 a_2) = 1/4,$$

for the a_3 allele must come from the mother and the a_2 allele from the father, F, and each of these occurs independently with probability $1/2$. The events or assumptions, all of which are *given*, will be separated by commas. Finally, although this is genetically less intuitive, there is no probabilistic difference between conditional events of the above kind and, for example,

$$P(\text{mother } M \text{ is } a_1 a_3 \mid \text{child } B \text{ is } a_2 a_3) = (1/2)p_1, \tag{6}$$

since again the segregation gives an event of probability $1/2$, while now the other allele whose population probability is required is the other allele of the mother, the a_1 allele.

This last assertion may become clearer when joint events are considered. The fact of several events all occurring, or occurring "jointly," is not conceptually difficult, but determining joint probabilities is seldom easy, although it is often a crucial step in computations. However, where the events are independent, the joint probability is easily determined as the product of the separate probabilities, for example,

$$P(M \text{ is } a_1 a_3, F \text{ is } a_1 a_2) = (2p_1 p_3)(2p_1 p_2) = 4p_1^2 p_2 p_3. \tag{7}$$

Where events are not independent, the use of conditional probabilities providing independent contributions is often the easiest way to determine joint probabilities; for example,

$$\begin{aligned}
P(B \text{ is } a_2 a_3, & M \text{ is } a_1 a_3, F \text{ is } a_1 a_2) = \\
P(B \text{ is } a_2 a_3 & \mid M \text{ is } a_1 a_3, F \text{ is } a_1 a_2) \, P(M \text{ is } a_1 a_3) \, P(F \text{ is } a_1 a_2) \\
& = (1/4)(2p_1 p_3)(2p_1 p_2) = p_1^2 p_2 p_3.
\end{aligned} \tag{8}$$

Note that if events are independent,

$$P(M \text{ is } a_1 a_3 \mid F \text{ is } a_1 a_2) = P(M \text{ is } a_1 a_3).$$

This is intuitively correct; being given the genotype of F does not alter the probabilities for the independent individual M. Another example is

$$\begin{aligned}
P(B \text{ is } a_2 a_3, M \text{ is } a_1 a_3) & = P(B \text{ is } a_2 a_3 \mid M \text{ is } a_1 a_3) P(M \text{ is } a_1 a_3) \\
& = (1/2)p_2 (2p_1 p_3) = p_1 p_2 p_3.
\end{aligned}$$

However, consistency requires that this joint probability is also

$$P(M \text{ is } a_1 a_3 \mid B \text{ is } a_2 a_3) P(B \text{ is } a_2 a_3),$$

which gives the conditional probability for M given B obtained in equation (6).

Often, joint events will be listed separated by commas, as in equations (7) and (8). Any underlying assumptions or hypotheses requiring specification will be listed similarly. Where the joint nature of a set of events is to be emphasized, the symbol & will be used, and should be read as "and." Mathematicians may prefer the equivalent set notation for intersection, $\cap$, but & is more easily recognized and understood for the type of events to be considered in this text. Only one "given" ($|$) can occur in a probability, and everything preceding it is to be conditioned upon all the events and assumptions that follow it. Thus,

$$P(B \text{ is } a_2a_3 \ \& \ M \text{ is } a_1a_3 \mid F \text{ is } a_1a_2)$$

means the probability for the genotypes of both M and B jointly, *both* being conditioned upon the genotype of F (although, of course, in this particular example M is independent of F in any case). The notation

$$P(B \text{ is } a_2a_3 \mid M \text{ is } a_1a_3 \ \& \ F \text{ is } a_1a_2)$$

would mean the probability of B being of type a_2a_3 given the genotype of both M and F. Generally, however, it is only for the events whose joint probabilities are required that the notation & is needed to emphasize this joint occurrence. Thus, for notational clarity, "&" will normally be used only for events preceding "$|$".

Finally, for completeness, consider the *union* of events; that is, instances when one or more of several events occur. In this text, these unions do not play an important role; the event "B is a_2a_3 or M is a_1a_3 or both" will be of little practical use. The event "B is a_2a_3 or a_1a_2" may be considered, but this is not a general "and/or"; rather, it is a case of mutually exclusive alternatives. For such unions, clearly, the probabilities sum;

$$P(B \text{ is } a_2a_3 \text{ or } a_1a_2) = P(B \text{ is } a_2a_3) + P(B \text{ is } a_1a_2).$$

There will be many instances in which events will be partitioned into mutually exclusive alternatives, and further details of the type of probability manipulation involved will be found in appendix 1, but the more general union of events will seldom be relevant.

1.9. Further reading

One of the most useful general introductions to human genetics is Stern 1973. The author's emphasis is on medical traits, but other aspects are covered as well, and to any newcomer to the subject, of whatever background, I recommend the book highly. Cavalli-Sforza and Bodmer (1971) give a thorough and clear introduction to the ideas of population genetics. The details of many blood-group systems are described, together with those of other systems important in the analysis of the characteristics of individuals and of populations. Ewens (1969) gives a concise account of basic population genetics which is rather more mathematical in style, but is clearly written. He includes a fuller account of the effects of linkage between two loci than can be given here. An account more closely related to the analysis of data on individuals is given by Li (1976), while Falconer (1981) provides a comprehensive approach to the analysis of quantitative traits. The last three texts provide a more mathematical background to the subject, but none demands mathematical or statistical expertise; rather, each provides a useful introduction to the ideas of data analysis in human genetics that is suitable for either the geneticist or the mathematician. More-advanced texts are those of Crow and Kimura (1970) and Jacquard (1974). These deal in more detail with some of the theoretical topics touched on in later chapters and will be referred to there. They also provide useful background material, but require more mathematical knowledge than is needed to follow the present text. No basic reading list would be complete without the four-volume work of Professor Sewall Wright (1968–78). Although his account is of the genetics of populations, and so does not impinge directly upon pedigree analysis, many of the sections on aspects of population structure are relevant (vol. 2, 1969), and the whole work provides important background for students wishing to pursue the subject in a wider context.

2. Gene Identity by Descent

2.1. Relatives and gene identity

This chapter deals with the basic genetic consequences of genealogical relationship, restricting attention mainly to straightforward family relationships: cousins, uncles, sisters, and so on. Genetically, attention is further restricted to a single Mendelian autosomal locus (section 1.2); every individual carries two genes, one received from his father and the other from his mother. The word *relatives* refers to blood relatives (individuals with common ancestors), and relationships are defined only within a specified genealogy over some limited time span. If an individual (*A*) and his uncle (*B*) are also second cousins (figure 4), this may be important; that they are also sixth cousins is unlikely to be so. Although individuals will be found to have common ancestors if their ancestry is traced back far enough, for our purposes they will be described as unrelated unless a precise relationship is specified.

For traits that are partially or wholly genetically determined, what is the basis of similarities between relatives? Why does one expect *A* to be more similar to *B* than to his unrelated uncle by marriage *C* or to his first cousin once removed *D*? Any given set of individuals may carry the same alleles; there are many copies of an allele in the population. However, relatives are more likely to do so, for they may carry copies of a single gene inherited from one common ancestor. For example, a rhesus-negative allele carried by *A* may derive from his grandmother *E*, who may have passed on this same gene to her son *B*. Genes that are copies of a single gene in a common ancestor of the individuals who now carry them are said to be *identical (by descent)*. Such identical genes must be of the same allelic type, while nonidentical ones may or may not be. The possibility of mutation, an event that changes the allelic type of a gene as it is passed from parent to child, is here ignored. Although mutation is a crucial evolutionary mechanism, probabilities of mutation are negligible within the limited time span of most of the genealogies considered in practice.

Thus, relatives are similar because they may carry identical genes More precisely, there are different combinations of genes in individuals which may or may not be identical. For example, *A* and *B* may receive identical genes from *E*. Further, *A*'s gene received from his father, *F*, may also be identical, all three genes deriving from the common grandfather *G* of *F* and *E*. Alternatively, *A*'s gene received from *F* may be identical to that received by *B* from *E*, but not to that received by *A* from his mother, *M*. In general, there are many possibilities, particularly when more than two indi-

Figure 4. The example genealogy discussed in the text

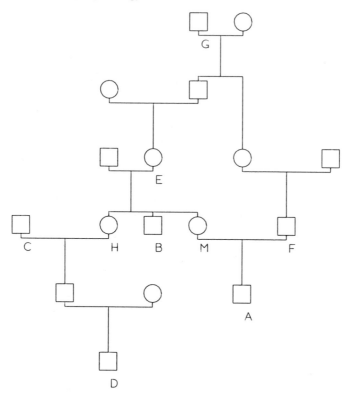

viduals, or more than one gene locus, are considered. Any genealogical relationship determines a probability for each possibility. Generally, closer relationships give higher probabilities for more of the relevant genes to be identical. For example, A and B have a higher probability of a gene in common than do A and D, while A and C have zero such probability because they have no common ancestor. These probabilities of the possibilities of gene identity are the basis of all the genetic consequences of genealogical relationship. In this chapter we shall be concerned with the specification of possibilities and the determination of probabilities. Only an elementary knowledge of probability is required; most of the derivations depend on simple counting arguments. For readers unfamiliar with the terminology of probability, some basic definitions and results are given in appendix 1.

Finally in this section, the ideas of degree and multiplicity of cousin-type relationships are introduced, since these will later provide useful examples. Between two individuals, the degree of their relationship deriving from a single ancestor or ancestral couple relates to the number of generations that separate the ancestor from the individuals. The smaller of the two generation counts gives the degree of a cousin-type relationship, the additional generational steps to the other being referred to as *removed*. Children of full sibs are first cousins. Thus A and D are, via E and her spouse, first cousins once removed. But F and E also are first cousins, via G and his spouse; thus A and H (the sister of B) are second cousins, and A and D are second cousins twice removed. Sibs are 0th cousins. Individuals with only one common parent are half sibs or half 0th first cousins, and corresponding to each cousin-type relationship there is a half-cousin one, when only one member of an ancestral couple is a common ancestor to both individuals.

Where there are several common ancestors, there may be simultaneously several cousin-type relationships, as for A and D above. Where these are duplicates of a single simple relationship, one has multiple-cousin relationships; the simplest example is double first cousins [figure 5(a)]. Here there are two duplicate first-cousin relationships between B_1 and B_2, via the

Figure 5. The multiplicity of first-cousin and half-first-cousin relationships: (a) double first cousins; (b) one-and-one-half first cousins; (c) three-halves first cousins; (d) four-halves first cousins (or quadruple half first cousins).

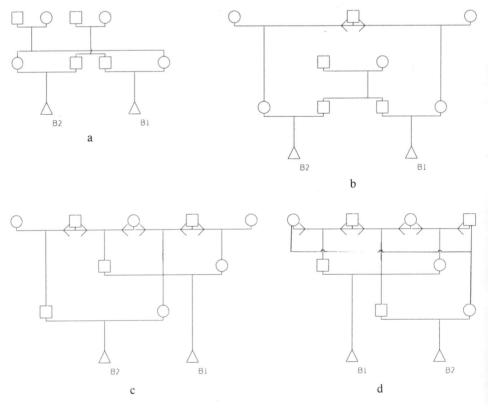

two separate pairs of common grandparents. Full- and half-cousin relationships may be combined; figure 5(*b*) shows one-and-one-half first cousins. Note that this is not the same as three-halves first cousins [figure 5(*c*)], a relationship that involves three separate half-first-cousin links. The maximum possible number of half-first-cousin links is four [figure 5(*d*)]: quadruple half first cousins will prove a useful example in section 2.4. This terminology may be extended to cousin relationships of more remote degree; for example, octuple half second cousins. However, it is not particularly illuminating to do so. In some texts first cousins once removed are referred to as one-and-one-half cousins, but this convention can cause confusion between the degree and the multiplicity of a relationship and will not be used here.

2.2. Genealogies

Although establishing the terminology for pairwise relationships is a useful preliminary to actually tracing a genealogy, it is also necessary to be able to specify a joint set of relationships such as those of figure 4. Since all relationships derive from parent-offspring links, specification of the two parents of every individual is sufficient to determine the complete genealogy. Unknown parents may be specified as 0, but if one parent of an individual is specified, then so must the other be; if only "*H* and *B* have mother *E*" is specified, it cannot be known whether *H* and *B* are sibs or half sibs unless the fathers also are assigned identification numbers. Then every individual either has no parent specified and is a *founder*, or has both parents specified and is a *nonfounder*. To encompass relationships more remote than parent-offspring, the missing individuals must be inserted. For example, *F* and *E* were previously specified only as first cousins via *G* and his spouse; now their four parents and common grandparents must be included in the specification of parent-offspring links.

Where other information on individuals is available, this may be added to the basic (individual, mother, father) triplet. In particular, sex and age (or year of birth) aid in checking the consistency of a genealogy. Consistency is taken to mean any genetically feasible collection of triplets, regardless of whether it includes demographically impossible features such as a grandson-grandmother mating. The only requirements are that every individual can be unambiguously assigned a sex and that no one is his own ancestor. Thus, the set of four triplets between eight hypothetical individuals labeled 21 to 28

$$25, 21, 22; \quad 26, 22, 23; \quad 27, 23, 24; \quad 28, 24, 21$$

is consistent, although it is clearer when written as

$$25, 21, 22; \quad 26, 23, 22; \quad 27, 23, 24; \quad 28, 21, 24$$

(with 21 and 23 as females and 22 and 24 as males, or vice versa). On the other hand, the three triplets

$$25, 21, 22; \quad 26, 22, 23; \quad 27, 23, 21$$

are not, since they cannot be rearranged so that 25, 26, and 27 each have a parent of either sex.

The second requirement of consistency is most easily checked by requiring an ordering of the listed genealogy in which every individual is preceded by his parents. Such an ordering is often computationally convenient. It is sometimes also convenient if founders head the list, but for other purposes it may be more efficient to assign them the last possible position so that they will not precede their descendants. The genealogy of figure 4 is redrawn in figure 6, the individuals now being assigned identification numbers in such a way that the natural ordering is the required one (table 4). More generally it will be necessary to have two sets of numbers, one assigned by the geneticist or anthropologist, used for all input and out-

Figure 6. The genealogy of figure 4, with individuals labeled so that the natural ordering is the required one

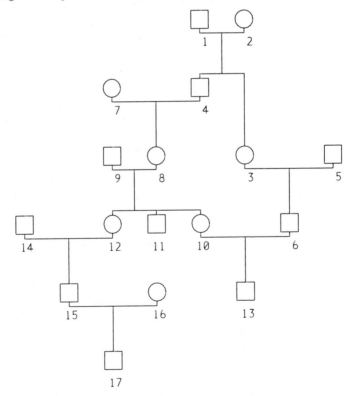

Table 4. Ordered listing for the genealogy of figure 6

Individual	Mother	Father	Sex (0 = female 1 = male)	Generation
1	0	0	1	0
2	0	0	0	0
3	2	1	0	1
4	2	1	1	1
5	0	0	1	0
6	3	5	1	2
7	0	0	0	0
8	7	4	0	2
9	0	0	1	0
10	8	9	0	3
11	8	9	1	3
12	8	9	0	3
13	10	6	1	4
14	0	0	1	0
15	12	14	1	4
16	0	0	0	0
17	16	15	1	5

put purposes, and the other entirely internal to the computer program, which relabels according to the ordering required. If dates of birth are available, it may be simplest to order the nonfounders by these, checking that each has a date later than the dates specified for his parents. If birth dates are unobtainable, it is convenient to assign individuals a generation number by which the nonfounders can then be ordered. This can be accomplished by starting from the founders (generation 0) and working repeatedly through the genealogy, assigning any individual both of whose parents are of already assigned generations a generation one greater than the maximum of these two. If this can be completed without contradiction, the genealogy is consistent in this respect.

All relationships are now defined via the set of triplets that constitutes the genealogy. For example, B_n ($n > 0$) is an *ancestor* of B_0 if there exist $B_1, B_2, \ldots, B_{n-1}$ such that B_{i+1} is a parent of B_i ($i = 0, 1, 2 \ldots, n - 1$). B is a *descendant* of B_0 if B_0 is an ancestor of B. Individuals are (genetically) *related* if they have a common ancestor. Individuals are termed *spouses* if they have a common offspring specified in the genealogy. This is clearly an abuse of everyday terminology, but this (nongenetic) relationship is of interest when, and only when, there are common offspring on whom there are genetic or further genealogical data. Individuals are *connected* if there is a chain of parent-offspring and offspring-parent

Figure 7. Alternative representations of genealogies: (*a*) parent-offspring links drawn for quadruple half first cousins; (*b*) the marriage node graph of the example genealogy; (*c*) a marriage node graph of quadruple half first cousins. Open squares and circles denote males and females, respectively, as previously. A marriage node is denoted by a circle circumscribing a square, and a branch point due to the multiple marriage of an individual is indicated by a circle within a square (whatever the sex of the individual).

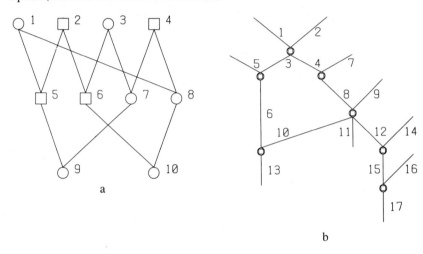

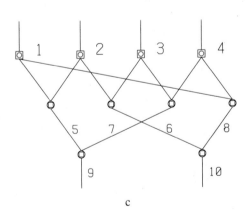

links from one to the other. They are *simply connected* if they have either a common ancestor or a common descendant. All the individuals of the example genealogy are connected, and indeed are simply connected.

The standard diagrammatic representation of genealogies was introduced in section 1.1, but it is difficult to represent complex relationships clearly in this way [see figure 5(*d*)]. Sometimes an improvement is obtained by representing each parent-offspring line directly rather than by connecting spouses [figure 7(*a*)]. This representation is more useful when tracing ancestral paths (see section 2.3 below), but for large and complex genealogies it is no simpler than the previous form. An alternative method is to represent marriages by points and an individual by a line connecting his parents' marriage to his own; figure 7(*b*) shows the example genealogy drawn in this way. Problems arise when an individual has several spouses, for then he must be represented by several lines—or better, a branching line [figure 7(*c*)]. This *marriage node graph* representation of genealogies greatly simplifies drawings of complex genealogies of several hundred individuals, such as will be encountered in later chapters. It also illuminates some computational procedures. However, for very large genealogies the picture is hardly less confusing in this form than in the traditional form, and the general optimal representation of genealogies remains an interesting unsolved problem.

2.3. Kinship and inbreeding

The two simplest probabilities of gene identity by descent are the classical kinship and inbreeding coefficients. The *kinship coefficient* $\psi(B_1, B_2)$ between two individuals is the probability (given only the genealogy and the fact of Mendelian segregation) that an autosomal gene chosen randomly from B_1 is identical to a homologous (same locus) one randomly chosen from B_2. Clearly this is the same for each autosomal locus, and $\psi(B_1, B_2) = \psi(B_2, B_1)$. An individual is *inbred* if his parents are related (within the specified genealogy). An inbred individual (B) has positive probability of having two identical genes at an autosomal locus. The probability of this event is the *inbreeding coefficient* $f(B)$ of individual B. Thus $f(B) = \psi(F_B, M_B)$, where F_B and M_B are the parents of B, for the two homologous genes of B *are* randomly chosen ones from his father and from his mother. Although the kinship coefficient is an insufficient characterization of pairwise relationship, it remains the single most useful one.

The efficient computation of inbreeding or kinship coefficients is a long-standing problem. Three methods will be demonstrated, not only because each can be useful, but more importantly because they exemplify the three general approaches to computations on genealogies. One class of methods derives from the original *path-counting* method of Wright (1922). A *path* from B_1 to B_2 is a chain of offspring-parent links from B_1 to a common ancestor A of the two individuals, followed by a chain of parent-off-spring links from A to B_2, with no individual occurring twice in the total chain. Although ancestors of A are also, in a sense, common ancestors of B_1 and B_2, the term *common ancestors* will be reserved for individuals A who are at the vertex of some path from B_1 to B_2 (figure 8). Consider B_1 and B_2 with single common ancestor A, who himself has two identical genes with probability $f(A)$. If A does not have two identical genes at the locus in question, the probability that he will pass identical genes to each of his two relevant offspring is $1/2$, while if he does, the probability is 1. Hence the overall probability is

$$(1/2)[1 - f(A)] + 1 \cdot f(A) = (1/2)[1 + f(A)].$$

If there are n and m segregations from A to B_1 and B_2, the probability that this gene will also first descend to each of the two individuals and then be the one chosen is

$$(1/2)^{(n-1)+(m-1)+1+1} = (1/2)^{n+m}.$$

Thus, if this is the only path of distinct individuals from B_1 up to a common ancestor and down to B_2,

$$\psi(B_1, B_2) = (1/2)^{n+m+1}[1 + f(A)].$$

Now, there may be several such paths, p, from B_1 to B_2 via the ancestor A, and, of course, there may also be several distinct common ancestors, each at the vertex of several paths each of distinct individuals. The crucial point of the argument is that the descent to and choice of the genes from B_1 and

Figure 8. Determination of common ancestors for computing kinship coefficients. The letter A denotes common ancestors of B_1 and B_2.

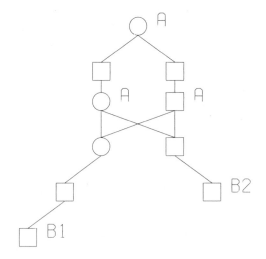

B_2 are, over different ancestors and different paths, mutually exclusive events (see appendix 1). The total kinship coefficient is thus simply the sum over different A's and p's;

$$\psi(B_1, B_2) = \Sigma_A \, \Sigma_p \, (1/2)^{n(A,p)+m(A,p)+1} [1 + f(A)],$$

where $n(A, p)$ and $m(A, p)$ are the n and m values for the ancestor A and path p.

For example [figure 9(a)], for quadruple half first cousins, each of the four grandparents is an ancestor A for one path with $n = m = 2$, and $\psi(B_1, B_2) = 4(1/2)^5 = 1/8$. The same is true for double first cousins [figure 9(b)]—the first indication that the coefficient of kinship is not a sufficient summary of a relationship. The case of an individual and his n^{th}-generation descendant is given by taking $m = 0$; this case must often be treated separately in genealogy computations, and the reader should convince himself that this is true. Finally, note that ancestors A may be related, or may even be ancestors of each other. The only requirement is that loops contributing to the inbreeding of an ancestor A should not be counted, but should be included in the factor $[1 + f(A)]$. In figure 9(c) there are thus four ancestors, giving a total of six paths and a kinship coefficient $3/8$ (table 5).

Although the path-counting approach is conceptually simple and is much used (Stevens 1975), it is not easily applied on genealogies of any complexity. Efficient identification of paths and ancestors is difficult. Further, path-counting methods are not easily extended to considerations of identity or nonidentity between more than two genes for it then becomes difficult even to characterize the mutually exclusive events, and this has led to some confusion in the literature.

Alternative methods rest on the basic equation

$$\psi(A, B) = (1/2)[\psi(M_A, B) + \psi(F_A, B)], \tag{9}$$

provided A is not B nor an ancestor of B, together with

$$\psi(A, A) = (1/2)[1 + f(A)] = (1/2)[1 + \psi(M_A, F_A)]. \tag{10}$$

Equation (9) results from the fact that a gene chosen from A is with probability $1/2$ a randomly chosen gene from F_A, and with the same probability a randomly chosen homologous gene from M_A, and the identity probabilities are then the kinship coefficients between F_A and B and between M_A and B. Subject to the proviso that A is not B nor his ancestor, the latter gene identities are independent of the segregations from M_A and F_A to A. Equation (10) has been encountered previously; $\psi(A, A)$ is simply the probability that two homologous genes independently segregating from A are identical. There are further standard equations that result from repeated application of (9). For example,

$$\psi(A, B) = (1/4)[\psi(M_A, M_B) + \psi(M_A, F_B) \\ + \psi(F_A, M_B) + \psi(F_A, F_B)], \tag{11}$$

Figure 9. Computation of inbreeding and kinship coefficients: (*a*) quadruple half first cousins; (*b*) double first cousins; (*c*) a complex example.

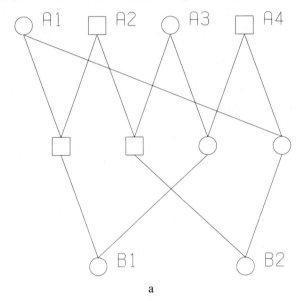

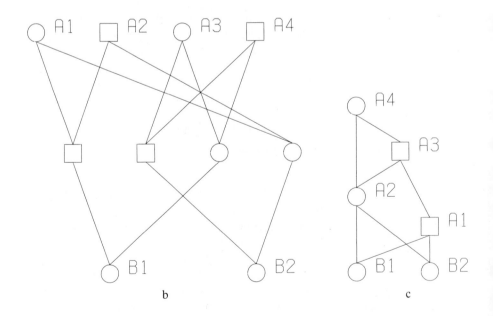

Table 5. Computation of the kinship coefficient for the genealogy of figure 9(c)

Vertex ancestor	Path*	n	m	$f(A)$	Contribution to ψ
A_1	$B_1 \underline{A_1} B_2$	1	1	0	$(1/2)^3$
A_2	$B_1 \underline{A_2} B_2$	1	1	$1/4$	$(1/2)^3[5/4]$
A_3	$B_1 A_1 \underline{A_3} A_2 B_2$	2	2	0	$(1/2)^5$
A_3	$B_1 A_2 \underline{A_3} A_1 B_2$	2	2	0	$(1/2)^5$
A_4	$B_1 A_2 \underline{A_4} A_3 A_1 B_2$	2	3	0	$(1/2)^6$
A_4	$B_1 A_1 A_3 \underline{A_4} A_2 B_2$	3	2	0	$(1/2)^6$
A_4	$B_1 A_2 \underline{A_4} A_3 A_2 B_2$ (not a path; A_2 is repeated)				

Note: Total kinship $\psi(B_1, B_2) = \dfrac{3}{32} + \dfrac{5}{32} + \dfrac{1}{8} = 3/8$.

*Underlining indicates the vertex of the given path.

provided A is not B nor an ancestor nor descendant of B. The latter equation will be of use in section 2.4, but normally use of the previous form (9) is most efficient. Note that (9) can always be applied either to A or to B, using the symmetry of kinship coefficients, unless A is B, in which case (10) applies.

There are two ways in which the above equations can be implemented. One is to start at the founders and work down the ordered genealogy (that given in table 4, for example), computing, storing, and then reaccessing the kinships as required. Individuals M_A and F_A precede A, and thus, at the stage of considering individual A, $\psi(A, B)$ may be computed for every B preceding A. Computationally this method is trivial, but the storage and reaccessing problems are horrendous on any large-scale genealogy. Unless all pairwise kinships are required repeatedly (for a detailed analysis of their distribution, for example), the method is not useful. It is introduced for its simplicity, and also as an example of what I shall term a *sequential* method, since the aim is to work sequentially through the genealogy. Such methods have sometimes been termed *recursive*, but they should be distinguished from the true recursive algorithms described below. They have also been termed *iterative* methods, since equation (9) is applied repeatedly, but this terminology could lead to confusion with methods in which a complete computation is repeated in order, for example, to obtain successively better estimates of unknown genetic parameters (section 6.4).

Given the advent of recursive block-structured computer-programming languages, equations such as (9) can be implemented precisely as they stand, for a routine can be defined implicitly (that is, by "calling itself"). Provided the MOTHER and FATHER arrays are previously set, the programming definition of a routine KINSHIP by

KINSHIP$[A, B] = (1/2)\{$KINSHIP$[$MOTHER$(A), B]$
$$+ \text{KINSHIP}[\text{FATHER}(A), B]\},$$

with appropriate alternatives if A is B or a founder, provides the result. The two arguments are reversed when necessary in order to expand always on the individual later in the ordered genealogy. Thus, to return again to the example genealogy, one might wish to compute $\psi(D, A) = \psi(17, 13)$. The program would make recursive calls as in figure 10, completing each branch from the top of the page before backtracking to the next. The degree of embedding gives the power of $1/2$ required in the contributions. Although figure 10 appears complicated, it is computationally by far the most efficient method when only a few pairwise kinships, or perhaps the inbreeding coefficients, are required. The procedure can be implemented on any ordered listing, but the late positioning of founders in the ordering is important to efficiency. For example, in figure 10, $\psi(16, 13)$ is recognized as 0 without tracing further ancestry, since 16 is a founder who cannot be an ancestor of the earlier-positioned 13. If many pairwise kinships are to be computed, another improvement in efficiency may be to store some of these and reaccess them when they are encountered in the ancestry of other pairs. However, the basic advantage of a recursive method is that it eliminates the requirement to store, although it does so at the expense of some recomputation and hence some inefficiency in terms of time. Another advantage of block-structured languages is that one can define structures that are a pair of integers (r, k) representing the numbers $r/2^k$ in the lowest possible terms, and specify all the standard arithmetic operations upon them. Exact probabilities can be computed on large and complex genealogies without the risk of rounding errors.

One final point is of interest. Kinship and inbreeding coefficients are probabilities and hence lie between 0 and 1. If inbred individuals are permitted, it is possible to construct an ancestry for two individuals such that their kinship coefficient is any specified $r/2^k$ in the open interval $(0, 1)$. This is intuitively clear, and has been widely recognized (Wright 1922), but a neat, explicit construction of such ancestry has been given recently by Karigl (1982). The genealogies may involve repeated matings of many descendants to the same ancestor, and so will not be of practical relevance in human genetics, but this idea that in the limit the whole closed interval [0, 1] is "attainable" by kinship coefficients, and hence also by inbreeding coefficients, will recur below.

2.4. A pair of noninbred relatives

Consider now a pair of relatives, neither of whom is inbred, although their parents may be so. Since neither of the two individuals can carry two identical genes, there are only three possibilities of gene identity (figure

Figure 10. An example of the recursive method for computing kinship coefficients. Each expansion to the mother (M) and father (F) of the first (higher-numbered) individual is shown as a branching, with the two components labeled M and F. The numerical label on each arrow gives the level of embedding of the recursive calls, and so determines the cumulative power of $1/2$ involved. Thus, the total kinship is computed as

$$(1/2)^5(1/2) + (1/2)^5(1/2) + (1/2)^8(1/2) + (1/2)^8(1/2) = 9/2^8 = 9/256.$$

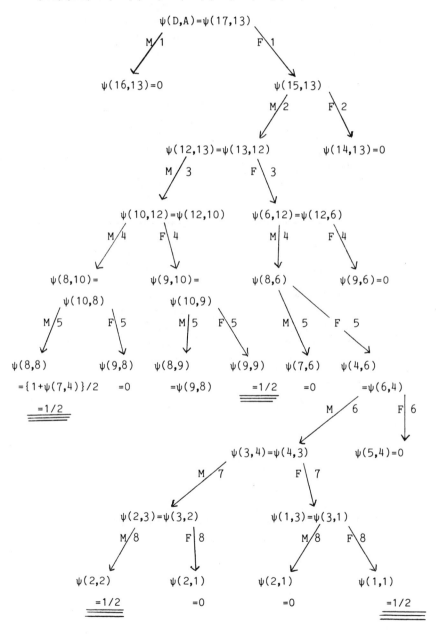

11): the individuals have two genes in common, or one, or neither. The probabilities of these events will be denoted k_2, k_1, and k_0, respectively ($k_2 + k_1 + k_0 = 1$). Consider first some examples:

(i)   *Unrelated*; there is no common ancestor and $k_0 = 1$.

(ii) *Parent-offspring*; the individuals are not inbred, so precisely the gene passed from parent to child is held in common and $k_1 = 1$.

(iii) *Half sibs*; provided the nonidentical parents are not related, the only common ancestor is the common parent A, who may be inbred. From the previous section, with probability $(1/2)(1 + f(A))$, A passes on identical genes to the two offspring. Thus, $k_1 = (1/2)[1 + f(A)]$ and $k_0 = (1/2)[1 - f(A)]$.

(iv) *Sibs with parents* M *and* F, *who may each be inbred but who may not be related*; sibs will have two genes in common if they receive the same gene from their mother and from their father; therefore, $k_2 = (1/4)[1 + f(M)][1 + f(F)]$. (The segregations in the two parents are independent events.) If the sibs receive the same gene from neither parent, they have no genes in common; therefore, $k_0 = (1/4)[1 - f(M)][1 - f(F)]$. Finally, $k_1 = 1 - k_2 - k_0$.

The above four examples provide the basis for other simple relationships, since these are made up from parent-offspring links descending from sib or half-sib ancestors. Each segregation introduces a factor of $1/2$ into the probability of gene identity. Thus,

(v)   *Uncle-nephew* [figure 12(a)]; since one parent of the nephew B_1 is unrelated, $k_2 = 0$. The uncle, B_2, will have a gene in common with B_1 if B_1's parent B_3 passes on a gene also held by B_2. If B_3 and B_2 have both genes in common, this will happen with probability 1; if only one, then the probability is $1/2$. Thus $k_1(B_1, B_2) = k_2(B_3, B_2) +$

Figure 11. Possible states of gene identity between two noninbred individuals: (*a*) both genes in common, probability k_2; (*b*) one gene in common, probability k_1; (*c*) all four genes distinct, probability k_0. The symbols 0, ×, \$, and % denote genes; the same symbols within each pair denote identical genes within individuals of the pair but not between pairs.

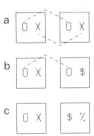

Figure 12. Examples of computation of *k*-probabilities showing typical segregation patterns of genes: (*a*) uncle-nephew (*M* and *F* may be inbred but not related); (*b*) parallel double first cousins. The symbols 0, ×, +, −, and $ denote genes, the repetition of symbols indicates genes that are identical by descent.

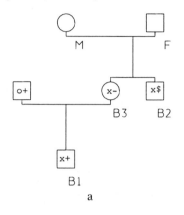

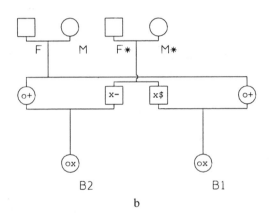

(1/2)$k_1(B_3, B_2)$, which, substituting for sibs B_3 and B_2 from (iv), reduces to $(1/2) + (1/4)[f(M) + f(F)]$, where F and M are the parents of B_2. Then $k_0 = 1 - k_1$.

(vi) *First cousins*; a further factor of 1/2 in the segregation from the uncle to his offspring gives $k_1 = (1/4) + (1/8)[f(M) + f(F)]$, where M and F are now the common grandparents. Again, $k_0 = 1 - k_1$.

Hence also

(vii) *Double first cousins*; write the above k_1 value for first cousins with grandparents M and F as $q(M, F)$, and consider parallel double first cousins (two sisters marrying two brothers) as shown in figure 12(*b*).

[Note that the probability $q(M, F)$ does not refer to any relationship *between* M and F]. Then the double first cousins have two common genes if they both receive the same gene from their fathers and the same gene from their mothers. Thus, $k_2 = q(M, F)q(M^*, F^*)$, where (M, F) and (M^*, F^*) are the two pairs of common grandparents. The double first cousins have no genes in common if they receive distinct genes from their mothers and distinct genes from their fathers; $k_0 = [1 - q(M, F)][1 - q(M^*, F^*)]$. Finally, $k_1 = 1 - k_0 - k_2$. If the common grandparents are not inbred, $q(M, F)q(M^*, F^*) = 1/4$ and $k_2 = 1/16$, $k_1 = 3/8$, $k_0 = 9/16$. Note that this is an extension of derivation (iv); the fact of independent segregations in nonintersecting ancestral paths is again used.

Further k probabilities for simple relationships can be found in any standard text (see section 2.8). They can be derived by direct arguments, such as those above, but they can also be derived via the coefficients of kinship, which can be computed by the methods described in section 2.3. Note first that for any pair of noninbred relatives

$$\psi(B_1, B_2) = (1/2)k_2(B_1, B_2) + (1/4)k_1(B_1, B_2), \tag{12}$$

for if the individuals have two common genes, then on drawing a gene from each there is probability $1/2$ of choosing two identical genes, while if they have only one common gene, the probability that this same one will be chosen from both the individuals is $1/4$ (figure 11). Also, from equation (11),

$$\psi(B_1, B_2) = (1/4)[\psi(M_1, M_2) + \psi(F_1, M_2) + \psi(M_1, F_2) + \psi(F_1, F_2)], \tag{13}$$

provided B_1 is not an ancestor nor a descendant of B_2. Finally, noninbred individuals have both genes in common if and only if they

> *either* receive the same gene from their mothers (M_1 and M_2) and from their fathers (F_1 and F_2),
> *or* receive the same gene from the opposite-sex cross-parent pairs (M_1, F_2) and (F_1, M_2).

Thus

$$k_2(B_1, B_2) = \psi(M_1, M_2)\psi(F_1, F_2) + \psi(M_1, F_2)\psi(F_1, M_2), \tag{14}$$

since the pairs of events are mutually exclusive, and the two within each pair are independent (appendix 1). The above three equations enable k_2, k_1, and $k_0 = 1 - k_1 - k_2$ to be determined for any pair of noninbred individuals, given the cross-parental kinship coefficients.

For relationships with $k_2 > 0$, it will normally be the case that the individuals are related

either via their mothers and via their fathers,
or the mother of each is related to the father of the other,
but not both.

Then only one of the two products in (14) is nonzero. For convenience, the case in which only the same-sex parent individuals are related will be considered. The second alternative clearly leads to equivalent results. Consider again, for example, the (parallel) double first cousins of derivation (vii). Here $\psi(M_1, M_2) = q(M, F)$, $\psi(F_1, F_2) = q(M^*, F^*)$, and $\psi(M_1, F_2) = \psi(F_1, M_2) = 0$. Hence $k_2(B_1, B_2) = q(M, F)q(M^*, F^*)$ and $\psi(B_1, B_2) = (1/4)[q(M, F) + q(M^*, F^*)]$. These equations give the same k_1 and thence the same k_0 as before. More generally, in terms of the kinship coefficients between the two mothers and the two fathers, this class of relationships gives

$$k_2 = \psi(F_1, F_2)\psi(M_1, M_2), \quad k_0 = [1 - \psi(F_1, F_2)][1 - \psi(M_1, M_2)],$$
$$\text{and } k_1 = 1 - k_0 - k_2.$$

Substituting these values into the expression $k_1^2 - 4k_0k_2$ yields

$$k_1^2 - 4k_2k_0 = [\psi(M_1, M_2) - \psi(F_1, F_2)]^2. \tag{15}$$

All relationships of this form must therefore satisfy $k_1^2 \geq 4k_2k_0$. However, since it is possible to construct a genealogy to provide any value of $\psi(M_1, M_2)$ and $\psi(F_1, F_2)$ between 0 and 1, any k-values satisfying this inequality and $k_2 + k_1 + k_0 = 1$ can be achieved.

In fact, it is possible for all cross-parental kinship coefficients to be nonzero, without the offspring being inbred. An example is quadruple half first cousins, where it is now assumed for simplicity that the common ancestors are not inbred. Here the mother (father) of each of B_1 and B_2 is half sib to both the mother and the father of the other, but the mother and father of B_1 (B_2) are not related to each other [figure 5(*d*)]. Thus, from derivation (iii),

$$\psi(M_1, F_2) = \psi(M_1, M_2) = \psi(F_1, F_2) = \psi(F_1, M_2) = 1/8.$$

Hence

$$\psi(B_1, B_2) = (1/4)(1/8 + 1/8 + 1/8 + 1/8) = 1/8,$$

and

$$k_2(B_1, B_2) = 2(1/8)(1/8) = 1/32.$$

Then

$$k_1(B_1, B_2) = 4\psi(B_1, B_2) - 2k_2(B_1, B_2) = 7/16,$$

and

$$k_0(B_1, B_2) = 1 - k_1(B_1, B_2) - k_2(B_1, B_2) = 17/32.$$

Note that for double first cousins,

$$k_2 = 1/16, \ k_1 = 3/8, \ k_0 = 9/16, \ \psi = 1/8;$$

for quadruple half first cousins,

$$k_2 = 1/32, \ k_1 = 7/16, \ k_0 = 17/32, \ \psi = 1/8;$$

and for half sibs,

$$k_2 = 0, \ k_1 = 1/2, \ k_0 = 1/2, \ \psi = 1/8.$$

There are thus many different relationships that have the same ψ but different (k_2, k_1, k_0); it is the latter that determine the joint distribution of genetic traits. Note, however, that the probabilities k_i are relevant to the individuals as a pair and are symmetrical between the two. A noninbred uncle-nephew pair can be genotypically distinguished from a parent-offspring pair, since each pair has different probabilities k_i and hence different pairwise genotype distributions. Within the pair, there is no genetic evidence as to which is the uncle and which the nephew, or which the parent and which the offspring. This symmetry can cause problems in the reconstruction of genealogies from genetic data (see section 3.5). In addition, there are different relationships that have the same (k_2, k_1, k_0). For example, for uncle-nephew as for half sibs, $k_2 = 0, \ k_1 = 1/2, \ k_0 = 1/2$, again now assuming no inbreeding in common ancestors. Grandparents also give the same k_i. Such relationships are not distinguishable on the basis of data on independently inherited genetic traits, each determined by a single autosomal locus.

This equivalence is, however, a feature of the genetic system considered. Grandparents, uncles, and half sibs are genealogically distinct relationships, and the probability k_1 is 1/2 in each case only as the effect of different numbers of different possible segregations leading to the same net result (figure 13). Consider instead two linked loci (section 1.6), with recombination fraction r. If $r = 0$, the two loci act as one, and the probability of a common gene at both (k_{11}, say) is 1/2. If $r = 1/2$, the two loci segregate independently, and k_{11} is $(1/2)(1/2) = 1/4$. Since there is no possibility of two common genes at a single locus for these relationships, and since for each locus separately $k_1 = k_0 = 1/2$, k_{11} provides a complete summary of the situation. For grandparent-grandchild, $k_{11} = (1 - r)/2$, since the genes received by the parent from the grandparent must be passed on without (further) recombination. For half sibs, $k_{11} = [r^2 + (1 - r)^2]/2 = R/2$, since whichever combination of genes is passed by the parent to the first child must also be passed to the second. The probability for the first locus is 1/2, and then for the other there may be recombination in the segregation to both offspring or to neither. Similarly, the combined expression, denoted R, will arise wherever segregation from a parent to two offspring is involved. For uncle-nephew, $k_{11} = [2(1 - r)R + r]/4$. This is

Figure 13. Three genealogically distinct pairwise relationships that are genotypically indistinguishable by data at unlinked autosomal loci: (*a*) grandparent-grandchild; (*b*) half sibs; (*c*) aunt-niece.

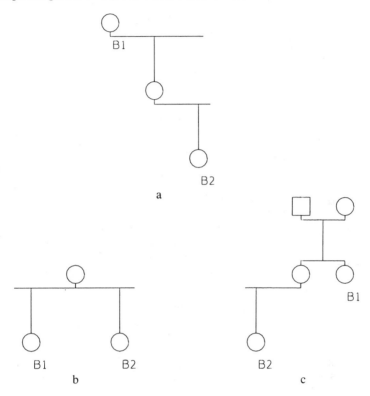

Figure 14. Probabilities of a gene in common at both of two linked loci, shown as a function of the recombination fraction *r* for each of the three relationships of figure 13. $P = k_{11}$.

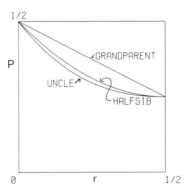

shown similarly by counting the possibilities. The term involving R expresses the probability that a common chromosome in the uncle and his sib will be passed without further recombination to the nephew. On the other hand, a recombination in the chromosome received by the nephew from his parent (probability r) results in his receiving a gene at one locus from his grandmother but at the other from his grandfather. The probability that his uncle received these same two genes (but obviously on different chromosomes) is then $1/4$. The second term thus comprises this possible combination of events. The three functions of r are shown in figure 14. They are, of course, distinct; the equivalence of the three relationships arises only when a single autosomal locus is considered. More complex genetic systems differentiate them, and in principle genealogical relationships are not equivalent unless they are so with respect to the total genome (see section 1.2). Nonetheless, in numerical terms the curves of figure 14 are similar. Even for linked loci, the two relationships have very similar phenotypic consequences. Moreover, a single autosomal locus is not merely a convenient mathematical artifact. It is a length of DNA sufficiently small that probabilities of recombination within it are negligible in the set of relevant segregations; the number of bases could be of the order 10^5, and include several functional genes whose joint effects are observed. Donnelly (1983) has considered the characterization of genealogical relationships in terms of lengths of DNA identical by descent, but two linked loci provide a simpler differentiation of the relationships of the current example.

Returning to the case of a single autosomal locus, points (k_2, k_1, k_0) with $k_2 + k_1 + k_0 = 1$ may be represented by points in an equilateral triangle of unit height, the k_i-values being the perpendicular distances of the point from the three sides. Figure 15 shows the representation of some of the above standard relationships in cases where the common ancestors are not inbred. The representation provides a heuristic picture of the similarities between relationships in terms of k-values, and hence in terms of expected genetic consequences. It is clear that sibs, parents, and monozygotic twins stand out as distinct from other relationships. There is, then, a group of "close relationships" down to perhaps first cousins. Relationships more remote than this are close to the "unrelated" vertex, and the genetic consequences of a single such pairwise relationship will be slight.

Finally in this section, consider a consequence of (12), (13), and (14) with some far-reaching implications. It is shown in appendix 2 that these equations imply

$$4k_2k_0 \leq k_1^2 \qquad (16)$$

for any relationship between two noninbred relatives. The area within the triangle that does not satisfy this restriction is also shown in figure 15. Equation (16) was deduced above [equation (15)] for relationships where only the same-sex parent pairs were related, but it holds also for the genea-

Figure 15. The space of identity state probabilities (k_2, k_1, k_0) between two noninbred individuals. The representation of a general point (k_2, k_1, k_0) with $k_2 + k_1 + k_0 = 1$ in the triangle is shown, together with the region excluded by the requirement $k_1^2 \geq 4k_0k_2$. Also shown are some standard relationships: $U =$ unrelated, $P =$ parent-offspring, $M =$ monozygotic twins, $FC =$ first cousins, $G =$ grandparent/half sib/uncle, $DFC =$ double first cousins, $S =$ sibs, $Q =$ quadruple half first cousins.

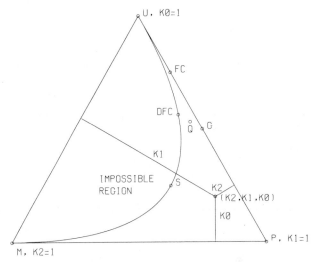

logically more general relationships such as quadruple first cousins. On the other hand, it was also seen that even the smaller class of relationships allowed all k-values satisfying (16) to be achieved. Thus, many different relationships must have the same k-values, and any possible such values can be explained by a relationship in which only the same-sex parent pairs are related. This will have implications in the estimation of relationships from genetic data (section 3.3).

2.5. Inbred relatives

When not only common ancestors but also the individuals themselves may be inbred, many more possible "states" of gene identity may occur at a single autosomal locus between the four genes of the two relatives. More precisely, there are fifteen such states (table 6), ranging from the case where all four genes are identical to that where none is identical to any of the others. However, these fifteen states subdivide the situations more finely than was done in the previous section; note that there are now seven states in which neither of the two individuals carries two identical genes. This is because states S_9 and S_{12} were previously grouped under the head "two common genes" with combined probability k_2, and states S_{10}, S_{11},

S_{13}, and S_{14} were all grouped under "one common gene" with probability k_1. The relationship between the seven states S_9–S_{15} and the cross-parental kinship coefficients of the previous section is considered in appendix 2, since it illuminates the restriction (16).

The detailed states $S_1, \ldots, S_{15}$ provide the fullest specification of the gene identity possibilities and arise naturally in probability computations via path-tracing methods. The coarser grouping does not distinguish the maternal and paternal origins of the two genes in an individual, but is a sufficient specification for the derivation of genotypic probabilities, since the genotype of an individual is the *unordered* pair of the allelic types of the two genes (section 1.2). Thus, the fifteen states reduce to nine classes of states (table 6), the states within each class being equivalent in their genotypic consequences.

For example, in discussing the genealogy of figure 4, in section 2.1 it was pointed out that A and B may have only common maternal genes via E (state S_{10}), or that the paternal gene of A may also be identical via G (state S_2), or that this last may be identical to the maternal gene of B, but not of A (state S_{13}). The first and third of these three possibilities are cases of precisely one gene in common between A and B. These states (S_{10} and S_{13}) provide the same joint genotype distribution (see section 2.6) and thus, when considering only individuals A and B, the two possibilities are equivalent. Only the sum of their probabilities is relevant. However, if A and B are considered jointly with other individuals, for example A's parents, one may then wish to distinguish the two states; the equivalence is not absolute but is relative to the problem and the set of individuals considered.

Note that in assessing the equivalences between states (table 6), the two individuals of the pair are distinguished. The cases in which the two genes of B_1 are identical to each other and to one of B_2's (the equivalent states S_2 and S_3) are *not* grouped into the same class as states S_6 and S_7, where the two genes of B_2 are identical to each other and to one of B_1's. This is because genotypic data are normally specified for an ordered set of individuals. Saying that B_1 has ABO blood type O and B_2 has blood type AB is not the same as saying that B_1 has type AB and B_2 has type O. Sometimes, however, genotypic data *are* unordered. For example, the relatives might be a pair (or more generally a set) of sibs, or of mutual first cousins, or simply a parent couple ancestral to other individuals, and the data might be that "one of the pair (or set) is affected and the other(s) not." For such a specification of data on a set of genealogically equivalent individuals, the probability of the event will not depend upon the ordering of the individuals, and further equivalences between the states may be introduced.

Computation of the probabilities of the states is a complex problem, for the joint descent to four genes must be considered simultaneously. For the example genealogy a direct derivation is possible for, in particular, the pair of individuals (A, B). Since E's spouse is unrelated to the other ances-

Table 6. States of gene identity between four genes, and distinguishable classes of states between two individuals

Individuals	B_1		B_2			
Genes	m_1	p_1	m_2	p_2	(maternal and paternal genes of B_1 and B_2, respectively)	
State: S_1	o	o	o	o	(1,1,1,1)	all genes identical
S_2	o	o	o	x	(1,1,1,2)	equivalent if maternal/
S_3	x	x	o	x	(1,1,2,1)	paternal origins of B_2's genes are disregarded
S_4	x	x	o	o	(1,1,2,2)	no common genes between individuals, but each has two identical genes
S_5	o	o	x	*	(1,1,2,3)	B_1 has identical genes
S_6	*	o	*	*	(1,2,1,1)	equivalent if maternal/
S_7	o	x	x	x	(1,2,2,2)	paternal origins of B_1's genes are disregarded
S_8	x	*	o	o	(1,2,3,3)	B_2 has identical genes
S_9	x	o	x	o	(1,2,1,2)	equivalent states;
S_{12}	*	o	o	*	(1,2,2,1)	two common genes
S_{10}	x	o	x	*	(1,2,1,3)	
S_{11}	o	x	*	o	(1,2,3,1)	equivalent states;
S_{13}	o	*	*	x	(1,2,2,3)	one common gene
S_{14}	o	x	*	x	(1,2,3,2)	
S_{15}	o	*	x	$	(1,2,3,4)	all genes distinct

Note: Each of the gene symbols (o, x, *, and $) denotes a single gene within a state, but no identity of genes bearing the same symbol between states is implied.

tors, the paternal gene of B can be identical only to the maternal gene of A. Further, if F and E do not have a gene in common, only states S_{10}, S_{11}, and S_{15} are possible. Thus, first consider the possibilities of gene identity in descent from G and his spouse to E and F, who are noninbred first cousins;

$$k_2(F, E) = 0, \; k_1(F, E) = 1/4, \; k_0(F, E) = 3/4.$$

In fact, the state that gives the common gene is S_{11}, since it is the mother of F and the father of E who are sibs, but this is not necessary to the derivation. Consider, then, the segregations down from E and F (figure 16); first, from F to the paternal gene A_p of A and from E to the maternal genes M_m and B_m of A's mother M and of B. These are then combined with the possible identities in the paternal genes of M and B, these being independent of the above identities, and, finally, the segregation from M to the maternal gene of A is incorporated. This gives eventually probabilities 1, 1, 1, 2, 29,

Figure 16. Computation of identity state probabilities for the example genealogy. Each symbol denotes a distinct gene *within* any set, but the same symbol does not indicate the same gene between different sets. Totals for states 2, 5, 12, 13, 15, 11, and 10 are, respectively, 1, 1, 1, 2, 29, 15, and 15 sixty-fourths, and the kinship coefficient is

$$[1 \times (1/2) + 1 \times 0 + 1 \times (1/2) + 2 \times (1/4) + 29 \times 0 + 15 \times (1/4) + 15 \times (1/4)] / 64 = 9/64.$$

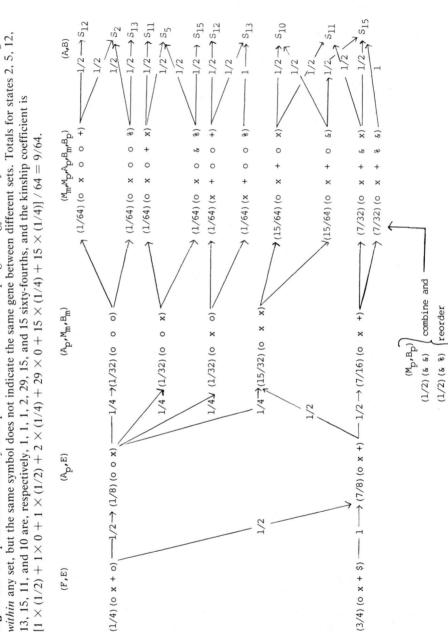

15, and 15 sixty-fourths, respectively, for the seven possible states S_2, S_5, S_{12}, S_{13}, S_{15}, S_{11}, and S_{10}. If distinction between equivalent states is not required, then the probability of states S_{10}, S_{11}, and S_{13} may be combined as $1/2$.

The above is a sequential derivation in the terminology of section 2.3. As will be shown in chapter 4, the procedure can be generalized, but its use is limited by the number of interlocking alternative paths of descent. Alternatively, Nadot and Vayssiex (1973) have implemented a path-counting method, but to obtain independent events whose probabilities can be combined (appendix 1), one must split the paths into nonoverlapping sections. This is a difficult task to automate in complex genealogies. Karigl (1981) has extended the recursive approach by defining "kinship coefficients" between more than just two genes. Such generalized kinship coefficients obey generalizations of the recurrences (9) and (10) of section 2.3 and so can be recursively implemented. There are, then, equations relating the state probabilities to these kinships, similar to (12) of section 2.4. This provides a neat general method for the present problem of four genes in two individuals, but more recurrence equations are required with each additional gene. Whereas for two genes there are the two recurrences (9) and (10), for four genes in two individuals a total of ten equations is required. On large genealogies the complexity and depth of the tree structure (figure 10) may become prohibitive. Although the computations required for analysis of complex genealogical relationships between two individuals can be effected by any of these three methods, in all three one encounters difficulties in considering identities between more than four genes (see also section 2.7).

2.6. Phenotypes of relatives

The present aim of characterizing relationships is to facilitate the analysis of observed genetic data, or the prediction of observable phenotypic events. In section 2.1 it was claimed that gene identity is the basis of similarities between relatives, and hence a fundamental component of the analysis of genetic data on genealogies. The precise relationship between gene identity and the joint probabilities of phenotypes of relatives is now demonstrated. For simplicity consider just a pair of relatives, as in previous sections.

Let H_1 and H_2 denote a pair of possible phenotypes for relatives B_1 and B_2 for a trait determined by the alleles at a single autosomal locus, and let $G_1, \ldots, G_m$ denote the possible genotypes at the locus. Then (see appendix 1) the probability of observing the specified phenotypes ("phen") can be partitioned into the probabilities under each possible pair of genotypes ("gen"):

$$P(\text{phen}(B_1) = H_1 \quad and \quad \text{phen}(B_2) = H_2)$$
$$= \Sigma_{i=1}^{m} \Sigma_{j=1}^{m} P(\text{phen}(B_1) = H_1, \text{phen}(B_2) = H_2, \text{gen}(B_1) = G_i,$$
$$\text{gen}(B_2) = G_j).$$

Or, abbreviating the notation,

$$P(H_1, H_2) = \Sigma_{i=1}^{m} \Sigma_{j=1}^{m} P(H_1, H_2, G_i, G_j),$$

which can be written

$$\Sigma_{i=1}^{m} \Sigma_{j=1}^{m} P(H_1, H_2 \mid G_i, G_j) P(G_i, G_j).$$

Further, since phenotypes are determined by individual genotypes, this reduces to

$$\Sigma_{i=1}^{m} \Sigma_{j=1}^{m} P(H_1 \mid G_i) P(H_2 \mid G_j) P(G_i, G_j). \tag{17}$$

The probabilities of phenotype given genotype, normally 0 or 1 for simply determined traits (section 1.3), are given by genetic characteristics of the locus such as dominance relationships between alleles. Thus, in order to determine the joint phenotype distributions of relatives, only a knowledge of these characteristics and of the joint genotype probabilities $P(G_i, G_j)$ is required.

So now let G_1^* and G_2^* denote any particular pair of genotypes for the ordered pair B_1 and B_2, who are in some genealogical relationship with total probabilities $q_1, \ldots, q_9$ for the nine genetically distinct classes of states now enumerated as in table 7. Then the probability of observing genotypes G_1^* and G_2^* for B_1 and B_2 can be partitioned into the probability under each of the nine mutually exclusive possible state-classes of gene identity;

$$P(G_1^*, G_2^*) = \Sigma_{c=1}^{9} q_c P(G_1^*, G_2^* \mid \text{state class } c). \tag{18}$$

The q_c are determined by the genealogy and do not depend on any genetic characteristics of the trait (other than Mendelian segregation at the locus). Thus, finally, probabilities $P(G_1^*, G_2^* \mid \text{state class } c)$ for each of the state classes c are required.

Now, in any state class c there are a certain number, r_c, of distinct genes $(1 \leqslant r_c \leqslant 4)$. Each distinct gene has some allelic type; all genes that are identical must have the same allelic type. Thus, the genotypes of B_1 and B_2 are determined by the allelic types of the r_c distinct genes. Assuming population frequencies $p_1, \ldots, p_s$ of alleles $a_1, \ldots, a_s$ $(\Sigma_{i=1}^{s} p_i = 1)$, the probability that a given gene is of type a_i is p_i and the types of distinct genes are independent. (Here population frequencies of alleles are interpreted as proportions in an infinite population pool from which the founders of the genealogy are chosen at random; see section 1.4.) Thus, the probability that the r genes of a given state take types $a_{j_1}, \ldots, a_{j_r}$ is

$$p_{j_1} p_{j_2} \cdots p_{j_r} \tag{19}$$

Table 7. Contributions of the classes of states to ordered genotype-pair probabilities

	1	2	3	4	5	6	7	8	9
Class of states	1	2	3	4	5	6	7	8	9
Previous states	S_1	S_4	S_2, S_3	S_5	S_6, S_7	S_8	S_9, S_{12}	S_{10}, S_{11} S_{13}, S_{14}	S_{15}
Probability	q_1	q_2	q_3	q_4	q_5	q_6	q_7	q_8	q_9
r_i	1	2	2	3	2	3	2	3	4
Genotype pair									
a_ia_i, a_ia_i	p_i	p_i^2	p_i^2	p_i^3	p_i^2	p_i^3	p_i^2	p_i^3	p_i^4
a_ia_i, a_ia_j	0	0	p_ip_j	$p_i^2p_j$	0	0	0	$p_i^2p_j$	$2p_i^3p_j$
a_ia_j, a_ia_j	0	0	0	0	0	0	$2p_ip_j$	$p_ip_j(p_i+p_j)$	$4p_i^2p_j^2$
a_ia_i, a_ja_j	0	p_ip_j	0	$p_ip_j^2$	0	$p_i^2p_j$	0	0	$p_i^2p_j^2$
a_ia_i, a_ja_k	0	0	0	$p_ip_jp_k$	0	0	0	0	$2p_i^2p_jp_k$
a_ia_j, a_ia_k	0	0	0	0	0	0	0	$p_ip_jp_k$	$4p_i^2p_jp_k$
a_ia_j, a_ka_l	0	0	0	0	0	0	0	0	$4p_ip_jp_kp_l$

Note: Subscripts $i, j, k,$ and l are all distinct.

and the total probability of genotypes G_1^*, G_2^* is, under the given state, the sum of these products over all combinations of allelic types assigned to genes resulting in the specified genotypes. Table 7 gives these contributions to the total probability.

For example, in the genealogy of figure 4, what is the probability that A is affected by a recessive trait, but that his uncle B is normal? First, we split the phenotypes into genotypes, knowing that the trait is recessive. Let a_1 denote the recessive allele, frequency p, and let a_2 denote any other alleles, total frequency $(1 - p)$. Then probabilities

$$P(A \text{ is } a_1a_1 \text{ and } (B \text{ is } a_1a_2 \text{ or } a_2a_2))$$
$$= P(A \text{ is } a_1a_1, B \text{ is } a_1a_2) + P(A \text{ is } a_1a_1, B \text{ is } a_2a_2)$$

are needed. Now, from the previous section we know that there are five possible classes of states of gene identity between A and B, namely, 3, 4, 7, 8, and 9, with probabilities as given in table 8. The probabilities of each of the two genotypic events under each of these states also are given in table 8, using (17). Thus, the total combined probability is as shown.

The above general derivation, and even the example, may seem unnecessarily long and complicated, but the aim has been to divide the problem into its separate components of genealogical relationship (q_i), population genetic characteristics (p_i), and trait characteristics (the phenotype-genotype relation), and to show how these combine to give the overall

Table 8. Computation of joint phenotype probability for individuals A and B of the example pedigree

Class of states	3	4	7	8	9
Representative states for (A, B)	$(\bullet\bullet\bullet\bigcirc)$ S_2	$(\bullet\bullet\bigcirc x)$ S_5	$(\bigcirc\bullet\bullet\bigcirc)$ S_{12}	$(\bullet\bigcirc\bigcirc x)$ S_{10}, S_{11}, S_{13}	$(\bullet\bigcirc x\$)$ S_{15}
r_i	2	3	2	3	4
Probability $\times 64$	1	1	1	32	29
Genotype-pair					
$a_1 a_1, a_1 a_2$	$p(1 - p)$	$p \cdot 2p(1 - p)$	0	$p^2(1 - p)$	$p^2 \cdot 2p(1 - p)$
$a_1 a_1, a_2 a_2$	0	$p \cdot (1 - p)^2$	0	0	$p^2 \cdot (1 - p)^2$

Notes: The a_1 allele has frequency p; the alternative, a_2, has frequency $(1 - p)$. The symbols $\bigcirc$, $\bullet$, x, and $\$$ each denote a single gene within each gene identity state.

$$\text{Total probability} = \frac{1}{64} \left[p(1 - p) + p(1 - p)^2 + 2p^2(1 - p) \right] + \frac{1}{2} p^2(1 - p) + \frac{29}{64} p^2(1 - p)(1 + p)$$

$$= \frac{1}{64} p(1 - p)[(2 + p) + 32p + 29p(1 + p)]$$

$$= \frac{1}{64} p(1 - p)(2 + 62p + 29p^2).$$

result. These same components will recur in our discussion of more complex genetic models (chapter 6) and more complex problems of computation on genealogies (chapter 4).

2.7. Arbitrary numbers of relatives

In this book, interest is not in relationships between only two individuals but in the joint set of relationships that exist in large and complicated genealogies. It remains the case that the genetic consequences of relationship are determined by the probabilities of the possibilities of gene identity by descent between the $2n$ genes of n individuals in any specified genealogy. But now there are vast numbers of possibilities and the probabilities are not easy to compute.

In theory, the ideas of the previous sections extend. Gene identity states can be counted and characterized, and so also the classes of states equivalent when maternal and paternal origins of genes are disregarded (Thompson 1974). This equivalence becomes of far greater practical importance, since it can result in a very great reduction in the number of probabilities to be computed. However, path-counting methods of determining the probabilities become infeasible. So also do recursive methods, although they extend in theory via Karigl's (1981) multiple kinship coefficients. The sequential methods to be described in chapter 4 can be used to determine probabilities of particular gene identity combinations of interest (Thompson 1980*a*), but the number of possible combinations is prohibitive. Another problem is that the attainable space of gene identity probabilities, not yet fully known even for two individuals, remains, for more than two, a completely unknown animal.

These extensions of the theory to arbitrary numbers of individuals provide a wide field of intriguing mathematical problems, and the interested reader may wish to pursue these via the references cited in this section. However, it is unnecessary to pursue them here, for fortunately one does not have to rely on gene identity probabilities in order to resolve the practical problems of computations on genealogies. Although the above description (2.6) of the relation between gene identity and phenotypic data remains valid, and is useful in providing a theoretical basis, it is not a sensible route for the analysis of phenotypic distributions. Indeed, although some of the results of this chapter will be used later, it may seem that little of the remainder of the text requires the detailed discussions given here. However, it should be recognized that gene identity underlies *all* studies of descent and ancestry via genetic data, and of the distribution of genetic traits among relatives. Even where it is not explicitly considered, it provides the basic theoretical justification of computational procedures and statistical methods.

2.8. Further reading

The outline of the theory of gene identity by descent given in this chapter is intended only to enable the reader to solve the simplest problems, to see the scope of the area, and to understand the elements of the theoretical framework underlying practical analyses of data on related individuals. The references that follow give far more detail of this framework. The first ideas of kinship and inbreeding were developed by Wright (1922) and extended by Cotterman (1940). The text by Crow and Kimura (1970) gives a clear account of these early developments. Gillois (1965) first fully characterized the general two-individual situation of fifteen states in nine classes, although Harris (1964) had previously used nine cases in approaching the problem of phenotypic correlations between relatives. This area is described in detail by Jacquard (1974; chap. 6), but note also the corrected approach to conditional phenotypic distributions given by Elston and Lange (1976). For a single autosomal locus, the more general theory of joint distributions on arbitrary numbers of individuals is considered by Thompson (1974) and by Cannings and Thompson (1981; chap. 2). The problem of characterizing the attainable space of gene identity probabilities was initiated by Thompson (1976c) and developed further by Thompson (1980b) and Karigl (1982). Gene identity by descent in more complex genetic systems has been considered by various authors. Some references to papers analyzing the case of two linked loci are given by Cannings and Thompson (1981); more recently, Donnelly (1983) has provided an analysis in which the genome is considered a continuum of DNA. To select just a few of the descriptions of various computational approaches, Nadot and Vayssiex (1973), Stevens (1975), Karigl (1981), and Thompson (1980a) give a varied and (between them) comprehensive coverage.

3. Estimating Relationships and Reconstructing Genealogies

3.1. The genetic structure of a population

Before returning to the subject of methodology (in chapter 4), let us consider one of three general problem areas of pedigree analysis, that of inferring genealogical relationships from phenotypic data. Since the joint phenotype probabilities of relatives are dependent upon the relationships involved, the observed joint phenotypes provide information about relationship. More precisely, the probability of observed phenotypes under a hypothesized relationship is the likelihood for that hypothesis. The likelihoods of alternative hypotheses can be compared, and hence, in principle, genealogies can be reconstructed. (For a basic introduction to likelihood principles and methodology, see appendix 3.)

A classic example of genealogical reconstruction from genetic data is paternity testing, where estimation of the relationship between a man and a mother-child pair is required. Most of the theory of paternity testing rests, however, on the probability that the man can be excluded from this relationship: exclusion probabilities have been considered for different genetic characteristics and under different true relationships of the man to the mother-child pair. Exclusion is possible in paternity testing because the child must have an allele in common with the true father at each genetic locus. For other relationships—for example, inferring sibs—definite exclusion is not possible, because there is positive probability that sibs will not share alleles at any particular locus. For example, an a_1a_2 individual cannot be the child of an individual with a_3a_3 genotype, since the parent must pass an a_3 allele to the child. If the parents were a_1a_3 and a_2a_3, the two could be sibs, although if the requisite parental genotypes are a priori improbable, the sib relationship is unlikely. In general, therefore, inferences must be based on relative likelihoods, or log-likelihood differences (appendix 3). Nonetheless, paternity testing is a useful example to bear in mind: the power to exclude individuals as parents is an important aspect of general reconstruction algorithms (section 3.5).

There are instances in which the reconstruction of genealogies from genetic data is a useful practical procedure. In many anthropological studies, where extensive data are collected, the genealogical data may be unreliable. Thus, the ability to check hypothesized relationships with genetic data can prove useful, if only to confirm the genealogy. In some instances the genetic data may even be the most accurate source of genealogical information; the case of some Amerindian data is considered in section 3.6. Reconstruction methods also have applications in small plant or animal populations. In other instances, the reconstruction of an accurately known genealogy from genetic data can be undertaken. An example is the genealogy of the Tristan da Cunhan population, considered for other purposes in chapter 5, or the genealogies of regular mating systems, which also have been considered in terms of genealogical reconstruction. Here the aim is not to infer new genealogical facts. Rather, it is that the ability to reconstruct a genealogy accurately is a measure of the genetic diversity in a population, and the errors in any reconstruction provide information on genetic similarities between different branches of the true genealogy. The attempt to reconstruct a known genealogy from genetic data can thus provide insights into the genetic structure of a population.

Although the theory aims at a detailed reconstruction of a genealogy, one if often more concerned that the estimate reflect the general characteristics of the genealogical structure than that it be accurate in detail. Thus, for example, one expects it to provide the correct distribution of sibship sizes; to reflect the true patterns of polygyny or remarriage, and the degree to which the sampled population is a complete, an isolated, or even a single genealogy; and to show the correct overall degree of relationship between groups of individuals. These aims are easier to fulfill, but less easy to assess, than a reconstructed genealogy that is accurate in detail. Methods for the general representations of population structures have been considered in many texts (for example, Jacquard 1974), but it is not clear which methods summarize the required features of a genealogical structure. One useful method is multidimensional scaling (or MDSCAL; appendix 4) of pairwise kinship coefficients or, in larger genealogies, of mean kinships between the sibships of the genealogy. Where genealogical information is available, the method can be applied to the actual kinships. With genetic data, it can be applied to estimated kinship or to kinship coefficients in a reconstructed genealogy. Similarities between the representations resulting from genetic and from genealogical data may be better indicators of success than, for example, the percentage of correct relationships inferred. Figure 17 shows the structure of a genealogy of 93 individuals in 20 nuclear families, and figure 18 illustrates the reconstruction of the same genealogy on the basis of simulated genetic data at 10 loci.

3.2. The theoretical framework

A genealogical relationship determines a set of probabilities over the classes of genetically distinguishable states of gene identity (chapter 2). These probabilities, together with the genetic characteristics of the trait in question, determine the phenotype distributions (see section 2.6). Conversely, therefore, given phenotypes for a number of traits whose genetic characteristics are known, the gene identity probabilities can be regarded as unknown parameters in the probability of observed phenotypes. This phe-

Figure 17. MDSCAL representation of a genealogy of 93 individuals in 7 groups of unrelated families. On the basis of mean kinship coefficients between sibships, the groups are well separated, and the structure of each group is clearly represented. A single founder is represented by a small square; each sibship, by a circle of radius proportional to the number of individuals therein. The lines show parental connections.

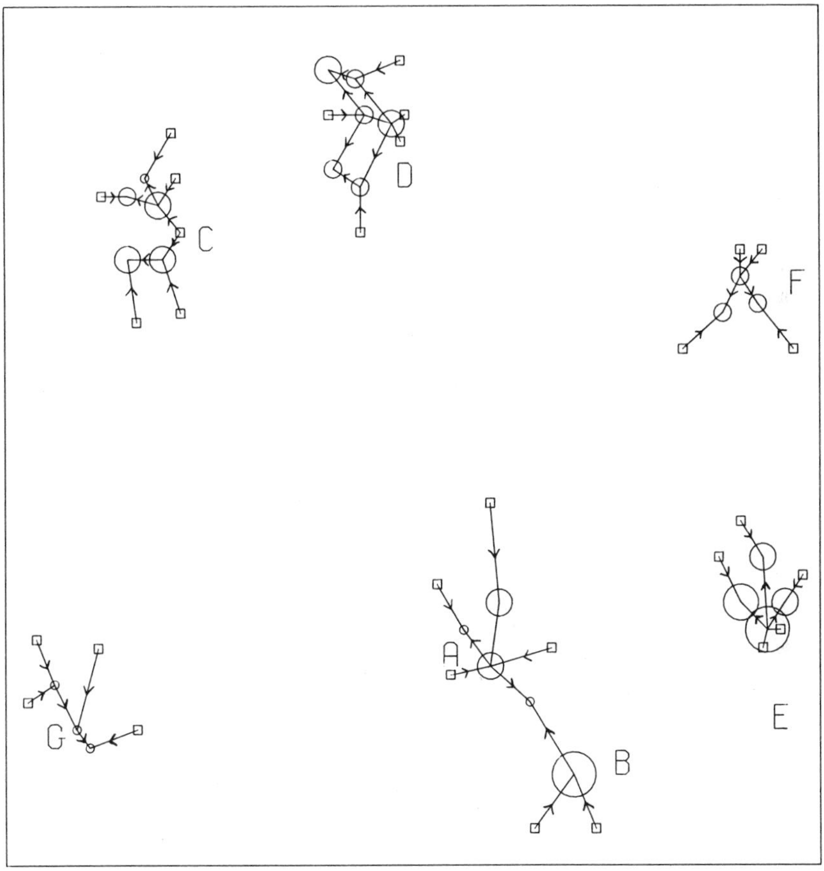

notype probability, as a function of the unknown gene identity probabilities, provides a likelihood for these parameters. If data for independently inherited (that it, unlinked) loci are available, each locus provides an additive contribution to the log-likelihood. By looking at data over a large number of loci, one may obtain accurate estimates of the parameters, for example, by using maximum likelihood (Appendix 3). Further, a measure of the information about relationships given by a genetic system is provided by the differences in log-likelihood between specified hypotheses to be expected

Figure 18. The same representation as figure 17, the input now being kinship coefficients in a genealogy reconstructed on the basis of genetic data at 10 (simulated) loci. For ease of comparison, one founder in each group is held at his previous position. Note the overall accuracy of the reconstruction; several groups are perfectly estimated, and, overall, 56 of the 64 nonfounders are correctly assigned to their parents. Note also, however, that the sibships of single individuals are not well determined; group *G* has largely been lost.

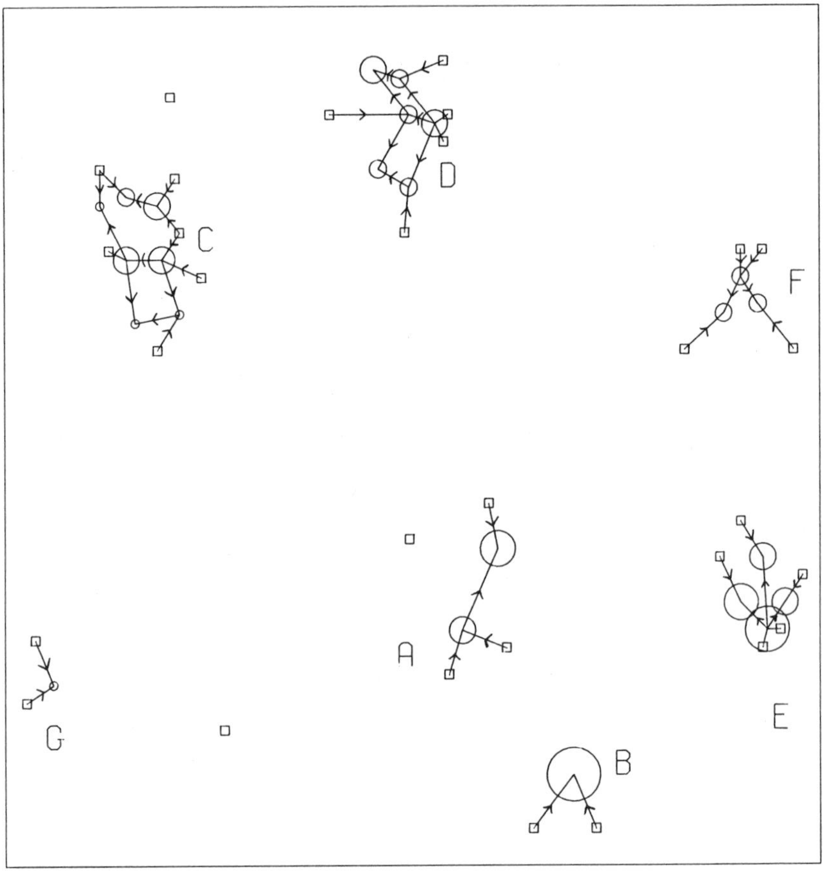

from data on that system. These expected log-likelihood differences are also additive over independently inherited loci.

The simplest situation is that of only one individual, in which case there are two possible states of gene identity. Either his two genes are identical by descent or not, with probabilities f and $(1 - f)$. That is, the inbreeding coefficient f (section 2.3) is the only parameter to be estimated from genetic data on the individual. The genotype probability at a single locus is

$$P(a_i a_i \mid f) = p_i [f + (1 - f)p_i]$$

$$P(a_i a_j \mid f) = 2p_i p_j (1 - f) \qquad (i < j),$$

where p_i is the population frequency of allele a_i [equation (2)]. These probabilities may be multiplied over independently inherited loci, giving a likelihood function for f. The maximum likelihood estimate of f is then that
value which maximizes this likelihood function. This example is given as an
introduction to the idea of likelihoods for gene identity state probabilities
rather than as a practical proposition. Although the procedure can be of use
for high levels of inbreeding (those obtaining in regular mating systems, for
example), it is well known that the power of phenotypic and even genotypic
data to detect the levels of inbreeding obtaining in most human genealogies
is slight (Yasuda 1968).

Since the phenotype probabilities are determined by the total probabilities of the classes of states, the probabilities of the separate detailed
states (section 2.5) can never be estimated from phenotypic data alone, nor
can relationships with the same probabilities of the state classes be distinguished. This means not only that uncle-nephew and half sib relationships
are indistinguishable (section 2.4) but also that in a parent-offspring relationship there is complete symmetry between parent and offspring. In the
reconstruction of extensive genealogies this can be a major stumbling block,
and in practice some age-ordering of the individuals is necessary to the
enterprise.

Note that the genetic characteristics of the trait must be assumed to be
known. These characteristics include not only dominance relationships between alleles but also population allele frequencies. In practice, in a study of
an isolated population, the allele frequencies may have to be estimated from
small samples, or even from the same interrelated individuals whose genealogy is to be reconstructed. The correct estimate of allele frequencies for
randomly chosen founders (section 1.4) is then unknown until the genealogy
is first reconstructed! Fortunately, the estimation of relationships is not sen-
sitive to small variations in the allele frequencies, and thus serious practical
problems seldom arise; a check may be made on the close similarity of estimated allele frequencies before and after reconstruction. Such an estimate
is, however, a source of variation in the analysis of real data, and should
lead to inferred relationships' being treated with more caution than the theory indicates.

3.3. Pairwise relationships

A case that can be usefully discussed in detail is that of inferring the
relationship between two noninbred individuals. Here the phenotype probabilities depend on the probabilities k_2, k_1, and k_0, of two, one, and zero
genes in common at the locus in question. The probability of a pair of phe-

notypes $(H_1^{(j)}, H_2^{(j)})$ at any locus j is linear in the probabilities k_i corresponding to the relationship between the individuals (see section 2.6);

$$P(\{H_1^{(j)}, H_2^{(j)}\} \mid \text{relationship} = k)$$
$$= k_2 P_2^{(j)}(H_1^{(j)}, H_2^{(j)}) + k_1 P_1^{(j)}(H_1^{(j)}, H_2^{(j)}) + k_0 P_2^{(j)}(H_1^{(j)}, H_2^{(j)}), \quad (20)$$

where $P_i^{(j)}(H_1^{(j)}, H_2^{(j)})$ is the probability of the phenotypes, given that the two individuals have i genes in common. Over s independently inherited loci the probability of phenotypes is the product of (20) over the loci;

$$P(\{(H_1^{(j)}, H_2^{(j)}); 1 \leqslant j \leqslant s\} \mid \text{relationship} = k)$$
$$= \prod_{j=1}^{s} (k_2 P_2^{(j)} + k_1 P_1^{(j)} + k_0 P_0^{(j)}), \quad (21)$$

where now for convenience the $(H_1^{(j)}, H_2^{(j)})$ are omitted. The maximum likelihood of estimate for k for the two individuals is that value of (k_2, k_1, k_0), subject to $k_2 + k_1 + k_0 = 1$, which maximizes (21) when the values of $P_i^{(j)}$ for the observed phenotypes are inserted. Note that the kinship coefficient $[\psi = (1/2)k_2 + (1/4)k_1$: equation (12)] cannot be estimated per se; it does not determine the pairwise distribution of characteristics.

Since the $P_i^{(j)}$ are nonnegative, the log of (21) is concave in k, and in general the log-likelihood has convex contours and a unique maximum (figure 19). Further, the true value of the relationship has maximum expected log-likelihood (appendix 3). The maximum likelihood estimate may be at a boundary point of the relationship triangle (section 2.4); indeed, for one locus it is necessarily at a vertex, and for two, at an edge. Nonetheless, over several loci a useful likelihood function is normally obtained. Further details may be found in Thompson (1975) or in Cannings and Thompson (1981; chap. 5). A problem arises with the restriction of genealogical relationships to the subset of the triangle (section 2.4). Since estimates of k not satisfying $k_1^2 \geq 4k_2 k_0$ are genealogically uninterpretable, estimates must be made within the restricted set. Due to these problems of interpretation of k-values, it is often preferable to compare the known k-values for standard simple relationships (parent, sib, cousin, etc.) and to distinguish only between these alternatives rather than maximize over arbitrary values of k.

There are two criteria, already referred to above, of the information potentially available in genetic data. The first is the probability of exclusion of a parent-offspring relationship (or parent-pair-offspring), this being more generally relevant as the probability of the existence of a sampled gene locus at which the individuals have phenotypes that do not allow for common alleles. This probability is of course dependent on the true relationship, but the basic value that determines all other is the one for unrelated individuals, who cannot share genes identical by descent. Only individuals without genes in common can be excluded as parent and offspring. Thus, for a general relative, at a single locus,

$$P(\text{exclusion} \mid k) = k_0 \, P(\text{exclusion} \mid \text{unrelated}). \quad (22)$$

An example is given in table 9; a locus with three equifrequent alleles at which genotypes are observable is considered. If the individuals are unrelated, the overall probability of a pair of genotypes at which there are no alleles in common iş given by $(1 \times 4 + 2 \times 1 + 2 \times 1 + 1 \times 4 + 2 \times 1 + 1 \times 4)/81 = 2/9$. If the individuals are in fact half sibs, it is necessary to consider the joint probabilities of the pair of genotypes tabulated in table 9, for the two individuals can no longer be considered independently. Summing these probabilities for the pairs that share no common allele gives a parent-offspring exclusion probability of $1/9$, verifying equation (22) (since here $k_0 = 1/2$) in this case at least.

The other information measure is the expected level of log-likelihood difference between alternative hypotheses of interest. This expectations depends not only on the relationship hypotheses to be compared but also upon the true relationship between the individuals. If the parent-offspring and monozygous-twin relationship are untrue, there is positive probability of genotypes for which $P_1^{(j)} = 0$ and $\log(0) = -\infty$. Thus, for this case, the expected log-likelihood of a parent (or twin) relationship is $-\infty$, and hence is not a useful criterion. For relationships that cannot be excluded, however, the measure is appropriate. Two particular values seem most useful: the expected difference in log-likelihood between half sibs and double first cousins, and between half sibs and sibs, in each case when the half-sib relationship is the true one. The first provides a measure of information along a line of constant kinship in the relationship triangle (figure 19); the other, information in an orthogonal direction. The example of table 9 also shows

Figure 19. The relationship triangle, showing standard pairwise relationships, the attainable region, and typical likelihood contours. The relationships G, $QHFC$, and DFC have the same coefficient of kinship.

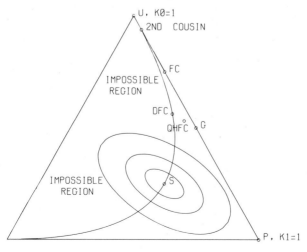

Table 9. An example of exclusion probabilities and log-likelihoods for a three-allele locus with equifrequent alleles

	a_1a_1	a_1a_2	a_1a_3	a_2a_2	a_2a_3	a_3a_3
Genotype of first individual						
Population probability or frequency ($\times 9$)	1	2	2	1	2	1
Total frequency of genotypes not sharing a common allele ($\times 9$)	4	1	1	4	1	4

Joint genotype probability if individuals are half sibs ($\times 162$):

Genotype of second individual		a_1a_1	a_1a_2	a_1a_3	a_2a_2	a_2a_3	a_3a_3
	$= a_1a_1$	4	5	5	1	2	1
	$= a_1a_2$	5	10	7	5	7	2
	$= a_1a_3$	5	7	10	2	7	5
	$= a_2a_2$	1	5	2	4	5	1
	$= a_2a_3$	2	7	7	5	10	5
	$= a_3a_3$	1	2	5	1	5	4

Log-likelihood for a relationship of double first cousins $+ \log(144)$:

Genotype of second individual ($\log 1 = 0$)		a_1a_1	a_1a_2	a_1a_3	a_2a_2	a_2a_3	a_3a_3
	$= a_1a_1$	$\log 4$	$\log 4$	$\log 4$	0	$\log 2$	0
	$= a_1a_2$	$\log 4$	$\log(10)$	$\log 6$	$\log 4$	$\log 6$	$\log 2$
	$= a_1a_3$	$\log 4$	$\log 6$	$\log(10)$	$\log 2$	$\log 6$	$\log 4$
	$= a_2a_2$	0	$\log 4$	$\log 2$	$\log 4$	$\log 4$	0
	$= a_2a_3$	$\log 2$	$\log 6$	$\log 6$	$\log 4$	$\log(10)$	$\log 4$
	$= a_3a_3$	0	$\log 2$	$\log 4$	0	$\log 4$	$\log 4$

how expected log-likelihoods are determined. The log-likelihoods for a double-first-cousin relationship are given for each genotype pair. These can be weighted by the joint half sib probabilities and summed to give an expected log-likelihood of

$$-\log(144) + [72 \log(4) + 12 \log(2) + 42 \log(6) + 30 \log(10)]/162$$
$$= -3.41,$$

were half sib the true relationship. Alternatively, they can be weighted by the product of the individual genotype probabilities to give an expected log-likelihood of

$$-\log(144) + [27 \log 4 + 12 \log(2) + 24 \log(6) + 12 \log(10)]/81$$
$$= -3.53$$

if the true relationship is that the two individuals are unrelated. In this subject area, natural logarithms are normally used (see appendix 3).

The data available in practice might normally consist of genotypes or phenotypes on perhaps fifteen reasonably informative blood-type, enzyme, or other marker loci. With this level of data, sib and parent relationships can be quite reliably inferred. They are well distinguished from each other, and from unrelated pairs of individuals. However, a parent or sib can sometimes be mistaken for a half sib or first cousin, or vice versa, and there is seldom power to distinguish these more remote relationships reliably from each other. Although the theory of this section extends to inbred individuals, and indeed to joint relationships between arbitrary numbers of individuals, the number of possible gene identity states makes this approach infeasible as a practical procedure. Instead, methods are required for the rebuilding of genealogies from the simple and most readily detected relationships, such as parent-offspring or sib.

3.4. An example of pairwise estimation

As an example consider again the genealogy from chapter 2. Hypothetical genotypic data for the individuals E, F, and their descendants and descendants' spouses are given in table 10. For easy reference the true pairwise genealogical relationships are given in table 11. Three sets of data are independently simulated in accordance with the characteristics of the loci specified in table 12. These characteristics are designed to be similar to those of loci available in blood enzyme-type studies from many populations. Normally, many more than seven loci should be available, so the combined set of twenty-one also is considered. On the other hand, some of the loci available in population studies may convey negligible information. Further, for simplicity, let us assume no dominance at the gene loci and independently inherited genes at different loci. These assumptions increase the available information.

No immediate conclusions are indicated by table 10; individual loci convey scarcely anything. Locus A3 shows an anomalous allele frequency, such as may arise in a genealogy where there are few independent genes. Loci B6 and C3 convey almost nothing, while locus B7 may be thought positively misleading as to the underlying genealogy. In fact, the data are as one would expect, given the locus characteristics, except that the most informative locus, 4, is in each case less informative than expected due to a chance excess of like allelic types among nonidentical genes. The pattern of this excess similarity leads to some anomalous estimates, which are discussed below. Table 13 gives the expected levels of information from the loci in terms of exclusion of parent-offspring links between unrelated pairs and of expected log-likelihood differences for true half sibs. Little information is to be expected from individual loci, and although the combined set is more encouraging, there is heavy dependence on the informative locus, 4.

On the basis of the simulated data, consider first the likelihood for the inbreeding coefficient, and the exclusion of parent-offspring relationships.

Table 10. Simulated genotypes on the example genealogy

Individuals (with identification numbers from fig. 6)

Locus	E 8	F 6	M 10	G 11	H 12	C 14	F* 15	M* 16	A 13	D 17
A1	12	11	12	12	11	11	11	13	11	11
A2	22	34	12	12	12	13	23	34	13	33
A3	22	12	12	12	22	12	22	12	22	12
A4	25	37	59	22	29	36	39	78	35	89
A5	12	12	12	22	22	11	12	11	22	12
A6	11	12	11	11	11	11	11	11	12	11
A7	33	34	13	13	13	34	34	24	13	34
B1	13	11	23	12	13	11	11	23	13	13
B2	14	12	12	12	12	23	12	12	22	12
B3	11	12	11	11	11	11	11	11	11	11
B4	79	77	57	79	79	39	39	18	57	13
B5	22	12	22	22	12	12	12	11	12	11
B6	12	11	11	11	12	11	11	11	11	11
B7	14	33	12	14	24	33	34	14	23	34
C1	11	33	12	12	13	11	13	13	23	13
C2	12	12	24	23	24	12	24	12	14	24
C3	11	11	11	12	11	11	11	11	11	11
C4	49	48	45	48	59	23	29	28	58	29
C5	11	12	11	11	11	12	12	11	12	11
C6	12	11	12	12	12	12	11	11	12	11
C7	23	12	13	13	23	13	13	24	11	14

Note: Each pair of digits denotes the pair of allelic types at the locus. $M*$ and $F*$ denote the parents of D; $F*$ is thus the child of C and H.

As expected, there is little information on inbreeding (table 14). The key individuals E and F have a greater than expected level of homozygosity, but only marginally so. Otherwise, all maximum likelihood estimates of inbreeding over all twenty-one loci are zero, apart from the truly inbred A [$f(A) = 1/32$]. However, log-likelihood differences are so small that no conclusions could possibly be drawn.

    Although over the sets of seven loci quite a few untrue parent-offspring links are possible, the parent-offspring exclusions do at least give some picture of the genealogy (table 15). Over all twenty-one loci virtually all untrue links are excluded. Yet even here the reader may want to try the following: write down all the possible parent-offspring links in random order, randomizing also the ordering of the two individuals within the pair. It is then not so easy to reconstruct the genealogy from this information alone!

Table 11. Specification of pairwise relationships
in the example genealogy

Relationship of		E	F	M	B	H	C	F^*	M^*	A
to	F	FC	—							
	M	P	RC	—						
	B	P	RC	S	—					
	H	P	RC	S	S	—				
	C	U	U	U	U	U	—			
	F^*	G	RC	G	G	P	P	—		
	M^*	U	U	U	U	U	U	U	—	
	A	G	P	P	G	G	U	FC	U	—
	D	FC	RC	FC	FC	G	G	P	P	RC

Note: FC = first   cousin/great-uncle/great-grandparent;   P = parent-offspring;
RC = remote cousin; S = sib; U = unrelated; G = grandparent/uncle/half sib.

Table 12. Genetic characteristics of the simulation loci

Locus A/B/C		1	2	3	4	5	6	7
Number of alleles		3	4	2	10	2	2	4
Allele frequencies (p_i)								
	1	0.50	0.30	0.85	0.10	0.60	0.75	0.25
	2	0.25	0.30	0.15	for each of 10	0.40	0.25	0.25
	3	0.25	0.30	—		—	—	0.25
	4	—	0.10	—		—	—	0.25
Individual heterozygosity ($1 - \Sigma p_i^2$)		0.625	0.720	0.255	0.900	0.480	0.375	0.750

The apparent clarity of the genealogy from the totals of table 15 is highly
dependent on the ordering of the individuals. It is also dependent on the
small number of individuals; even in a set of 100 there will be many more
possibilities, even if the exclusion probability for each unrelated pair is
high. On the other hand, the high degree of relationship between the individuals of the present example decreases exclusion probabilities [equation
(22)]. In a larger population the mean k_0, and hence the mean exclusion
probabilities, will be higher.

Table 16 presents the pairwise likelihood results. The log-likelihood
differences for the maximum likelihood relationship relative to the true one
are given for each of the sets of seven loci and for the combined set. For the
combination of twenty-one loci the log-likelihood difference relative to "un-

Table 13. Information characteristics of the simulation loci

Locus A/B/C	1	2	3	4	5	6	7
Parental exclusion probability	0.195	0.292	0.032	0.657	0.115	0.070	0.328
Expected log-likelihood G:DFC	0.0044	0.0070	0.0008	0.0245	0.0020	0.0014	0.0079
Expected log-likelihood G:S	0.0918	0.1194	0.0357	0.2175	0.0541	0.0466	0.1284

Combined characteristics of sets of seven loci and of the combined set of 21:

	7 loci	21 loci
Mean total heterozygous loci	4.105	12.315
Exclusion probability	0.895	0.999
Exclusion probability excluding locus 4	0.694	0.971
Exclusion probability for sibs	0.360	0.738
Expected log-likelihood G:DFC	0.048	0.144
Expected log-likelihood G:S	0.693	2.080

Note: In this and the following tables, all numerical values involving logarithms use natural logarithms, as is usual in this subject area (see appendix 3).

Table 14. Likelihoods for the inbreeding coefficient

	Individual									
Set	E	F	M	B	H	C	F*	M*	A	D
A	0.16	−0.10	−0.11	0.13	0.10	0.04	−0.05	−0.08	0.08	−0.01
B	−0.06	0.20	−0.05	−0.04	−0.12	0.03	−0.05	−0.06	−0.03	−0.06
C	−0.01	−0.02	−0.09	−0.11	−0.08	−0.08	−0.08	−0.06	−0.04	−0.06
Combined set	0.11	0.08	−0.25	−0.02	−0.10	−0.01	−0.18	−0.20	0.01	−0.13

Note: Log-likelihood differences between an inbreeding coefficient, f, of 0.02 and zero inbreeding ($f = 0$) are shown for the three groups of loci A/B/C and for the combined set.

related" also is given, this being the log-likelihood for the detection of any relationship against the null alternative. Parent relationships P are well distinguished when true, although there is a tendency for other relationships to be inferred as parent-offspring when the latter is not excluded. The lack of information on lines of constant kinship if noticeable. Sibs S may be confused with parents ($\psi = 1/4$), but not normally with anything else; half sibs G are often confused with double first cousins DFC ($\psi = 1/8$). The remote relationships, RC, which are close to the unrelated vertex U of the relation-

Table 15. Number of loci in each set which exclude a parent-offspring relationship between pairs of individuals

	E	F	M	B	H	C	F*	M*	A	D
E	—	2	+	+	+	2	1	3	1	2
F	1	—	2	2	2	0	0	0	+	1
M	+	2	—	1	0	1	0	3	+	1
B	+	1	0	—	0	2	1	4	1	2
H	+	1	0	0	—	2	+	4	1	1
C	2	1	3	1	1	—	+	1	1	1
F*	0	1	3	0	+	+	—	1	0	+
M*	2	3	2	2	1	3	2	—	3	+
A	2	+	+	1	0	1	1	2	—	1
D	2	1	3	2	1	0	+	+	1	—
E	—	1	+	+	+	1	0	1	3	1
F	4	—	1	1	1	2	1	0	+	1
M	+	5	—	0	0	1	1	2	+	1
B	+	4	1	—	1	1	1	1	1	1
H	+	4	0	1	—	1	+	1	1	1
C	5	3	5	4	4	—	+	1	2	0
F*	1	2	4	2	+	+	—	1	1	+
M*	6	3	7	7	6	5	4	—	1	+
A	6	+	+	3	2	4	2	6	—	1
D	5	3	5	5	3	1	+	+	3	—

Note: True parent relationships are shown as +. Upper tableau gives locus set A above the diagonal, locus set B below. Lower tableau gives set C above the diagonal, and grand total below.

ship triangle (figure 19), also are not well distinguished. There is, however, quite good power to distinguish four overlapping groups of relationships: nuclear family relationships (P, S), close relationships (FC, G, DFC), remote relationships (FC, RC), and individuals effectively unrelated (RC, U). For the sets of seven loci, estimating between these seven alternatives, 61 of 135 cases provide the correct maximum likelihood estimate. There are also a further 28 within-group estimates, giving overall 66 percent accuracy. For the combined set of twenty-one loci, 25 of 45 estimates are correct and 12 more are within-group, giving 82 percent accuracy. The (P, S) relationships are clearly detected by the log-likelihood differences relative to U. The (FC, G, DFC) group give smaller values, but are usually also quite well distinguished. In fact, most of the errors over the twenty-one loci are attributable to an anomaly in the data which is sufficiently marked to be noted by the simulation program. This is the close similarity of F to the two unrelated

Table 16. Estimation of pairwise relationship on the average genealogy: Maximum likelihood relationship ($\hat{R}$) and log-likelihood differences relative to true relationship (T) and to unrelatedness (U)

Pair	True relationship	Set A $\hat{R}$	$S(\hat{R}) - S(T)$	Set B $\hat{R}$	$S(\hat{R}) - S(T)$	Set C $\hat{R}$	$S(\hat{R}) - S(T)$	Total $\hat{R}$	$S(\hat{R}) - S(T)$	$S(\hat{R}) - S(U)$
E, F	FC	RC	0.038	FC	0	FC	0	FC	0	0.357
E, M	P	P	0	P	0	P	0	P	0	7.191
E, B	P	P	0	S	1.454	P	0	P	0	7.161
E, H	P	P	0	S	0.714	P	0	P	0	9.414
E, C	U	FC	0.144	U	0	DFC	0.394	RC	0.147	0.147
E, F^*	G	S	0.362	P	0.221	P	0.020	G	0	2.292
E, M^*	U	U	0	U	0	RC	0.006	U	0	0
E, A	G	DFC	0.075	U	0.584	U	2.014	RC	1.325	0.271
E, D	FC	FC	0	U	0.544	FC	0	U	0.248	0
F, M	RC	U	0.191	FC	0.066	U	0.025	RC	0	0.022
F, B	RC	U	0.166	G	0.364	DFC	0.223	RC	0	0.340
F, H	RC	RC	0	RC	0.113	U	0.079	RC	0	0.278
F, C	U	P	2.205	DFC	0.852	U	0	DFC	1.429	1.429
F, F^*	RC	P	2.354	DFC	0.392	RC	0	DFC	1.360	2.171
F, M^*	U	P	2.206	U	0	P	2.388	DFC	1.056	1.056
F, A	P	P	0	P	0	P	0	P	0	7.673
F, D	RC	S	0.936	RC	0	RC	0	FC	0.149	0.443
M, B	S	S	0	P	0.462	S	0	S	0	6.988
M, H	S	P	0.808	P	1.176	S	0	P	1.938	7.630
M, C	U	U	0	U	0	RC	0.005	U	0	0
M, F^*	G	P	0.846	U	1.435	DFC	0.513	DFC	0.484	0.482

Pair										
M, M*	U	U	0	DFC	0.054	U	0	U	0	0
M, A	P	P	0	P	0	P	0	P	0	8.036
M, D	FC	G	0.097	U	0.586	DFC	0.160	RC	0.158	0.057
B, H	S	P	0.335	S	0	U	2.346	S	0	4.684
B, C	U	U	0	FC	0.172	U	0	U	0	0
B, F*	G	FC	0.005	P	0.896	U	1.162	FC	0.141	0.447
B, M*	U	U	0	DFC	0.055	U	0	U	0	0
B, A	G	DFC	0.070	FC	0.012	FC	0.074	G	0	1.107
B, D	FC	U	0.220	U	0.431	U	0.506	U	1.156	0
H, C	U	FC	0.144	RC	0.002	U	0	RC	0.015	0.015
H, F*	P	P	0	P	0	P	0	P	0	7.152
H, M*	U	U	0	U	0	U	0	U	0	0
H, A	G	S	1.173	P	0.637	G	0	DFC	0.324	3.639
H, D	G	G	0	U	0.367	S	0.671	DFC	0.231	2.233
C, F*	P	P	0	S	0.782	P	0	P	0	7.958
C, M*	U	FC	0.119	U	0	FC	0.099	U	0	0
C, A	U	G	1.150	G	0.259	U	0	FC	0.743	0.743
C, D	G	S	0.515	P	0.666	P	0.021	G	0	2.183
F*, M*	U	FC	0.166	U	0	FC	0.187	RC	0.095	0.095
F*, A	FC	P	1.985	RC	0.015	FC	0	G	0.629	2.199
F*, D	P	P	0	P	0	S	1.521	S	0.250	10.970
M*, A	U	U	0	U	0	U	0	U	0	0
M*, D	P	P	0	P	0	P	0	P	0	6.695
A, D	RC	G	0.400	FC	0.017	FC	0.053	G	0.294	0.765

Note: The abbreviations for relationships or as in table 11, with the addition of DFC = double first cousin.

spouses C and $M*$, which gives excess similarity of F (and hence A) to that branch of the genealogy (including D, who is unexpectedly dissimilar from the family E, M, and B).

In practice more information is likely to be available than is provided by any one set of seven loci, but not often more than the combination. Overall trial-and-error might enable quite an accurate genealogy to be reconstructed from table 16, but without some age-ordering of the genealogy it again cannot be determined which of a pair is the grandchild and which the grandparent, nor indeed whether they are instead half sibs. To reconstruct a genealogy from separate pairwise inferences might be an intriguing game, but not a useful practical procedure. The pairwise relationships imply joint relationships between several individuals, such as offspring–parent-pair triplets or sets of sibs. There is more power to infer these relationships jointly than to infer component pairs, although the latter are useful in restricting the set of joint relationships that one might want to consider. As indicated above, a method of sequential reconstruction is required, building on the most readily distinquishable nuclear family relationships and including information on age-ordering.

3.5. Reconstruction; a practical algorithm

When a sample consists of a population of closely interrelated individuals, the reconstruction of its genealogy must incorporate both genealogical and demographic restrictions. In the first category may be placed such trivial observations as that a child cannot have two mothers, even if two women give maximum likelihood to the parent-offspring relationship. Further, in most human populations sibs are more common than half sibs. It is useful, therefore, to seek not only likely parent-offspring links but also parent pairs and sets of offspring. The second category includes restrictions on polygamy or incest, which may be considered demographically unlikely to have occurred in the particular study population. Yet such events may on occasion have substantial genetic likelihoods, and cannot always be ruled out.

Consider a "genealogy" of unrelated individuals; this is not a plausible hypothesis, but is a convenient base point for reconstruction. Its likelihood is the total product of all the population probabilities of all phenotypes over individuals and unlinked loci:

$$P(\text{data} \mid \text{all unrelated}) = \Pi_h \Pi_{j=1}^s P(\text{data on individual } h \text{ at locus } j).$$
(23)

A hypothesized genealogy may be specified as a set of nuclear families, i, with mother M_i father F_i and children C_{ih} ($h = 1, \ldots, n_i$). If genotypic data are available for all individuals, the likelihood of this hypothesis is the product of founder genotype probabilities mulitplied by the probabilities of genotypes of offspring (C_{ih}), given those of parents (M_i, F_i) for all hypothesized nonfounders:

$$\Pi_{j=1}^{s} \, [\Pi_{\text{founders}} \, P(\text{data on founder at locus } j)$$

$$\Pi_{\text{nonfounders}} \, P(\text{data on individual} \mid \text{parent data})]. \qquad (24)$$

Both (23) and (24) thus partition into multiplicative factors attributable to each locus, each family, and each child within the family. Then, in the log-likelihood difference between the nuclear-family genealogy and the base point of unrelatedness,

$$\log \left[\text{expression (24)} \right] - \log \left[\text{expression (23)} \right],$$

the terms corresponding to the founders cancel, leaving only those for each specified offspring. The net result is the sum of additive contributions:

$$\Sigma_{j=1}^{s} \Sigma_i \Sigma_{h=1}^{ni} \, \log \{ P(G_j(C_{ih}) \mid G_j(M_i), G_j(F_i)) / P(G_j(C_{ih})) \}, \qquad (25)$$

where $G_j(B)$ denotes the genotype of individual B. Thus, to reconstruct a genealogy of maximum likelihood, mutually compatible nuclear families providing large values of (25) must be found.

There are several practical difficulties in achieving this objective. First, in a population of even 200 individuals there are likely to be many possible parent pairs for each individual, and the genetic symmetry of the parent-offspring relationship makes age data essential. Children not only cannot be arbitrarily assigned to the most individually likely parent-pairs, but even when reconstructing by whole sibships, acceptance of one family can preclude acceptance of another. Clearly, large sibships will tend to provide the largest values of (25), but feasible sibship size is limited. On the other hand, these large hypothesized sibships do often include the true ones, in addition to offspring from elsewhere. Thus, in reconstruction the sibships can be accepted only provisionally, and the extra "sibs" must then somehow be weeded out. These extra "sibs" may sometimes be half sibs; some allowance for polygamy and second marriages must be made.

If incest is to be precluded, two offspring members of an already inferred nuclear family cannot be freely accepted as spouses; one must be removed from that sibship. In this direction, the choices are easy to program and the log-likelihoods of the alternatives are easy to compare. It is more complicated to restrict the acceptance of already inferred spouses as sibs. The practical solution to this problem has therefore been to consider groups of hypothesized mothers in decreasing order of age, so that sibships of the older generation are reconstructed first.

Although sibships are reconstructed as a whole, individual offspring must then be permitted to "move" to subseqently reconstructed families if this provides a higher likelihood. This movement is necessary to remove the extra offspring from unacceptably large sibships, to detect and reconstruct the smaller ones, and to reduce bias toward the mothers first considered. On the other hand, movement must be restricted if unacceptable levels of polygamy and polygyny are not to be inferred. In practice, various algorithms have been employed; the most successful has been to transfer offspring (if this provides higher likelihood) only to new sibships that are reconstructed on the basis of other individuals as yet without assigned parents. The disadvantage of this procedure is that single-child families are often not inferred. Due to the consideration of potential mothers in decreasing age order, and the fact that the younger ones have the smaller incomplete families, there is a bias against these women in the reconstructed genealogy. It is also clearly insufficient to consider only two-parent nuclear families; parents may be unavailable. Thus, in the final adjustments to inferred families, single-parent and no-parent sibships also must be considered, particularly, of course, among the older individuals, whose parents most likely have not been sampled.

Despite the ad hoc character of the above procedures, the combination of genetic and demographic information which they employ has allowed accurate reconstruction of several real and simulated genealogies of about 100 individuals. A part of the Tristan da Cunhan genealogy has been very accurately reconstructed from data on only seven genetic loci. The level of information available from the twenty-one hypothetical loci of the previous section is more than adequate. In view of the rather limited power with respect to accurate pairwise estimation, the method of joint sequential reconstruction is very successful. The case of an Amerindian study, where the true genealogy is perhaps not accurately known, is discussed below.

Consider first, however, the basis of the above procedure. Sets of individuals are assigned to those potential parents who provide the maximum value of (25). Thus, rather than determining the maximum log-likelihood relationship between a given set of individuals, the individuals who provide maximum likelihood increase on acceptance of a given relationship are sought. The former is a well-specified problem with a well-defined parameter space to which the statistical theory of maximum likelihood estimation will apply (sections 2.5 and 3.4, appendix 3). For the latter, however, there is no reason to suppose that *between individuals* true parents will provide maximum log-likelihood increase (25). Indeed, it can be shown that monozygous twins are, in this sense, always the "most likely parents," but this not a practical problem, since monozygous twins are unlikely to be mistaken for parent and offspring! However, it can also be shown that at two-allele loci with dominance, sibs can provide a higher expected value of (25) than do true parents, and that conditional on the nonexclusion of the sib as a parent, the same is true for many other genetic systems (Thompson 1976b.) Of course, given consistency of relationship estimation, they must provide still higher expected log-likelihood to the true sib relationship. Nonetheless, this finding reemphasizes the necessity for age data, the desirability of multiallelic loci, which can exclude more sibs as possible parents, and the necessity of considering sib hypotheses, at least to confirm the reconstructed genealogy. It also shows that the method is highly dependent not only on the likelihood considerations of the previous sections but also on the special exclusion-probability feature of the parent-offspring relationship.

3.6. An Amerindian genealogy

Several attempts have been made to reconstruct genealogies from real or simulated genetic data. One of the more practical but less successful attempts is described here, in order to illustrate both the surprising power of genetic data in very unpromising circumstances and the practical problems that can arise. Between 1965 and 1975, extensive genetic and anthropological studies were made of the Yanomama Indians of the Amazon rain forest, by J. V. Neel and others of the Department of Human Genetics, University of Michigan.[*] This work is reviewed by Neel (1978). In particular, a group of three interrelated villages (designated 03A/B/C) was studied intensively. Genetic data for all available individuals were collected; in fact, for 81, 43, and 59 individuals, respectively.

Genetic data for twelve genetic systems were available, including seven polymorphic loci with (effectively) codominant alleles (table 17). Although the data for the 183 individuals were not complete, it is a far more detailed and extensive study than is normally available for such a population. Genealogical and demographic data also were collected, although ages could only be estimated, and genealogical information may be unreliable. The possibility of reconstructing genealogical relationships from genetic data is therefore of practical interest in this population. As a preliminary data set, 96 individuals specified by the genealogical data as members of 48 offspring-parents triplets $(C; (M, F))$ were selected. These triplets will be referred to as the "putative" relationships. For the seven genetic systems used, 40 of the 96 individuals did not have complete data, but for 33 of these, information was missing at only one locus. The allele frequencies used in likelihood computations were the crude frequencies in the set of 183 individuals from the three villages. Table 17 shows that only three of the loci are highly informative. Age data are given in table 18.

The unreliability of genealogical data for the Yanomama is well known. High levels of polygyny and the often temporary nature of marriage relationships cause confusion to anthropologists and possibly also to the individuals themselves. Using only reliable genetic systems, exclusion of paternity had previously been reported in 6 percent of putative triplets, repre-

[*]I am grateful to Professor J. V. Neel for allowing me access to the data of section 3.6 during a visit to his department in 1975, and for permission to reproduce here some of the results of my work on them.

Table 17. Genetic systems used in analysis of Amerindian data, and estimated allele frequencies

System	Number of alleles	Allele frequencies				Parent-pair exclusion probability
MNSs	4	0.034	0.534	0.043	0.389	0.3553
Rhesus (C and E)	4	0.155	0.773	0.071	0.001	0.1778
Duffy	2	0.668	0.332			0.4645
Haptoglobin	2	0.874	0.126			0.1118
Gc	2	0.961	0.039			0.0127
PGM1	2	0.933	0.067			0.0357
Albumen: Yan2	2	0.907	0.093			0.0652
					Overall:	0.7756

Table 18. (Putative) age and age-difference distributions for the 96 individuals constituting 48 offspring–parent-pair triplets

Age or age difference	Nonfounders		Founders		Mother-offspring	Father-mother (counted for each offspring)
	Male	Female	Male	Female		
< 0	—	—	—	—	—	3
1–4	10	9	—	—	—	12
5–14	8	10	—	—	2	17
15–20	1	5	1	3	13	14
21–25	2	1	1	8	14	—
26–30	2		—	4	8	2
31–40	—	—	6	6	11	—
41–50	—	—	8	4	—	—
51–60	—	—	4	2	—	—
60+	—	—	1	—	—	—
Total	23	25	21	27	48	48

senting (since not all errors are detectable) an underlying error rate of 9 percent. Exclusions of putative maternity also were encountered. Among the 48 triplets among the 96 individuals in the three intensively studied villages, no less than 13 were excluded; 4 by the Duffy system, 2 by PGM, 3 by Rhesus, 2 by MNS, 1 by the Yan2 albumen polymorphism, and 1 due to possibly overrestrictive use of estimated ages by the reconstruction algorithm. A fourteenth individual was excluded by systems not used in the analysis, and three of the other exclusions were endorsed by exclusions at other loci. Although some of the exclusions could be due to genetic mistypings (the Duffy-*b* in particular being deemed unreliable) several of the putative relationships must be untrue. This raises the problem of criteria for judging a reconstructed genealogy; deviation from putative relationships is not necessarily evidence of error!

In addition, three of the putative triplets gave negative contributions to the log-likelihood of equation (25); this event is very improbable for a true triplet, and the likelihood criteria will clearly never detect such an instance, the hypothesis of unrelatedness being preferred. For example, for the Tristan da Cunhan data, only one putatively true relationship gave negative value, and only 1 percent of all possible links. For the Amerindian data the latter proportion was 25 percent, and the distribution of values was found to have been severely distorted by the missing data. When only the four loci for which all 96 individuals were tested were used, the proportion of possible links with negative log-likelihood fell, although of course exclusion probabilities and mean log-likelihood values also fell. However, even then the same three putative links, and also the one excluded outside the seven systems used, gave negative values. Although this could be due to the chance occurrence of high heterozygosity in the parents, there is considerable doubt as to the truth of these four links. Thus, in all, 17 of the 48 putative triplets are not inferrable from genetic data, leaving 31 triplets in 22 sibships which may be true and could be inferred.

Turning to the detection of triplets $(C; (M, F))$, table 19 shows that 3 individuals have more than 22 possible fathers, and that each of 11 females are mother-members (M) in possible triplets with more than 25 different males as the F member. One woman is the M member on triplets involving 53 different offspring. More usually, the younger individuals have around 20 possible fathers, and the older women have at least 20 possible offspring, and often a total of more than 200 $(C; (-, F))$ combinations. The possibilities are presented in this form because it is easier to construct demographically acceptable genealogies by considering mothers than by considering fathers. The biological and social constraints are tighter, and, given even approximate age data, a set of offspring is more easily identified as joint children of a female than of a male.

The power of the genetic data to exclude triplets is slight; there are approximately 20 older males, 20 older females, and 40 younger individuals, providing 16,000 potential triplets. Table 17 shows that 77 percent of triplets of unrelated individuals should be eliminated by the genetic data; in fact, there remain 4,264 genetically feasible ones. To identify the 31 putatively true ones will not be easy! A major problem is that sibship sizes are small: of the 29 putative mothers of the original 48 offspring, 15 have only one child, and 11 more only two. On the other hand, of the 31 inferrable triplets, 25 were included within the 10 most likely triplets for that mother,

Table 19. Genetically possible triplets among 96 individuals, 31 of whom are mothers in such triplets

Number k	Number of individuals with k possible fathers; total over possible mothers	Number of possible mothers with possible offspring by k different men	Number of possible mothers with k possible offspring; total over possible fathers of such offspring
0	7	—	—
1	16	1	1
2–3	9	—	1
4–7	7	—	2
8–13	10	—	2
14–17	17	1	3
18–20	12	4	3
21–23	15	5	3
24–25	—	9	3
26–27	3	11	—
28–33	—	—	4
34–39	—	—	3
40–43	—	—	5
53	—	—	1
Total	96	31	31

and 10 of the putative sibships were subsets of one of the 3 most likely offspring sets for that mother.

In the initial reconstruction of the genealogy the total log-likelihood increase [expression (25)] was 620.14, but only 3 of the 31 triplets were correct. In addition, however, 12 offspring were assigned to the putative mother (M) and 4 to the putative father (F). The total number of sibships inferred was 25, with a total of 61 offspring assigned. All save one of the putative nonfounders were assigned, but 14 putative founders were also; section 3.4 showed that parent-offspring links, if not excluded, are often preferred to true alternatives. When the 31 inferrable triplets were imposed, the maximum likelihood genealogy assigned 58 offspring in all, but had a log-likelihood of only 499.85, a vastly lower value. By a variety of procedures for transfer of individuals between sibships, a genealogy including 4 putative sibships with log-likelihood 623.30 was found. However, one including 9 putative sibships and additional 7 putative M and 1 putative F had log-likelihood not much smaller (619.52). Although $9+7=16$ (out of 31) correct M and only $9+1=10$ correct F may seem to be low rates of accuracy, combining triplet inferences enabled a section of genealogy including the putative relationships of 25 individuals over three generations to be correctly inferred.

It is noticeable that in all reconstructions the number of "correct" mothers exceeded the number of "correct" fathers. This not only demonstrates the information provided by biological restrictions, but also probably indicates the inaccuracy of the putative fathers and the possibly greater accuracy of genetically based inferences. In particular, three paternities that gave significantly larger log-likelihood than the putative ones contribute quite largely to differences in log-likelihood. On the other hand, in a closely interrelated population, close relationships of alternative fathers can lead to high variability in likelihood, and untrue triplets of high expected log-likelihood.

Overall, this study shows that high exclusion probabilities for untrue parents are essential if one is to reconstruct a genealogy accurately. Large sibships also help. Where these do not obtain, or where the genealogy includes many unsampled parents and unconnected individuals, many more relationships will be inferred than in fact hold. Nonetheless, even with the low level of genetic data here, the inferred relationships should at least include many true ones. The fact that the genetic data on 96 individuals permit more than 4,000 $(C; (M, F))$ triplets shows how inadequate these data are. Yet these same data give rise to likelihoods allowing detection of a reasonable proportion of putative relationships. The unique maximum likelihood estimate of genealogy is not useful, even where it can be determined, but the true links are almost always among the most likely, and links common to a wide class of likely genealogies are often reliable inferences.

3.7. Phenotypic data

The above methodology and examples deal only with the use of genotypic data at unlinked loci. The vast array of systems now available for study, the increased resolution of phenotypes, and especially the "codominant alleles" of DNA data and restriction enzyme polymorphisms mean that ample genotypic data will be available in the future. The main practical development of the methodology required may be the use of linked loci. This does not create theoretical problems; two linked loci jointly provide a likelihood for a pairwise or joint relationship through their joint segregation. Since many haplotypes (combinations of alleles at several loci on a single chromosome) may be identifiable, the power of data at groups of closely linked loci to distinguish genealogical relationships will be high. Evaluation of the likelihoods may involve heavy computation, but the methods of this chapter all extend in principle to a set of s unlinked groups of loci, each j in equations (20) through (25) now denoting a complex of several linked loci.

It is important, however, that best use be made of studies already carried out, and attention therefore cannot be restricted to loci at which genotypes are observable. Also, in reconstructing genealogies, there will always be relevant unsampled individuals whose genotypes can never be known. For example, in inferring sib relationships in the absence of the parent-pair the likelihood implicitly involves those parental genotypes. Of course, the theory of estimation of gene identity state-class probabilities (sections 3.2, 3.3) is not restricted to genotype data, and for pairwise estimation (sections 3.3, 3.4) there is little difficulty in computing likelihoods under phenotypic rather than genotypic data. In principle, likelihoods for relationship could be computed even on the basis of quantitative traits, although results would be heavily dependent upon the assumed model for the determination of the trait, and the power to distinguish relationships would be very slight.

There are two areas where difficulties arise with phenotypic data. One is the study of information and expected log-likelihoods. The effects of specific simple dominance patterns can be numerically evaluated, but a general assessment of the loss of information due to inaccurate knowledge of genotype is more complicated. The second area is the reconstruction of extensive genealogies (3.5), where the log-likelihood can only be separated into contributions from separate nuclear families where genotypes of all "connecting" individuals common to two families are known. For phenotypic data, inferred nuclear families can no longer simply be combined in order to build up a genealogy, and even computation of the likelihood becomes difficult (see section 4.6). The possible nuclear families interact not only via demographic and social factors but also via genetic ones. Acceptance of two families on the basis of phenotypes may imply underlying genotypes for the common individuals which are even inconsistent. More generally, the overall likelihood may be much less than the sum of the contributions, owing to the different underlying genotype distributions implied by the separate relationships, but there is no simple formula. The basic problem is thus again inaccurate knowledge of genotype from phenotype.

Both problems can therefore be studied as aspects of the *EM-algorithm*, which is a method for maximizing likelihoods and also studying their properties when certain information that ideally one would like to have (here, knowlegde of the genotypes) is unavailable. Dempster, Laird, and Rubin (1977) first gave a general theoretical discussion of this class of problems, but the method has long been recognized in practical applications (Smith 1957). Thompson (1983*a*) discussed it in relation to problems involving likelihoods on genealogies. The idea is that likelihood estimates can be obtained by reconstructing the unavailable variates as their expectations, given the actual data and hypothesized parameter values, and then making likelihood estimates on the basis of these reconstructed variables. Then, since these estimates will affect the expected values of the unavailable variates, the procedure is repeated until convergence is obtained. More details of this iterative procedure and its convergence properties can be found in the references cited.

In principle this method can be used in algorithms for rebuilding genealogies as follows: Acceptance of a nuclear family determines a probability distribution for the genotypes of the members. The genotype probabilities for a "connecting" individual may then be incorporated as "data" in considering the likelihood for the connecting family, and acceptance will modify the distribution for peripheral members of both families. For most genetic systems, effects beyond the immediate nuclear family will be slight, and in practice the method can be quite successful. However, computation is a lengthy process, and as yet only small genealogies have been considered in this way. The method is subject to the disadvantage that acceptance of a likely family at an early stage could have far-reaching effects on the overall genealogy reconstructed, and further investigation of the properties of this procedure is necessary.

3.8. Further reading

All the statistical analyses in this book will use the likelihood approach to statistical inference. Although the basic definitions required are given in appendix 3, readers who are unfamiliar with the approach may find it useful to consult Edwards (1972) for a far fuller yet accessible discussion. The idea of reconstructing genealogies was first presented by Edwards (1967), but this area has not been explored by many authors. Specific questions, such as estimation of the inbreeding coefficient, have been considered (Yasuda 1968), while Jacquard (1974, sec. IV) discusses measures of distance between individuals on the basis of genetic data. The theory of pairwise estimation is given by Thompson (1975), but the practical procedures of Thompson (1976a) are limited to genotype data, and the "paradox" problem of Thompson (1976b) remains unresolved. More details and discussion are given by Cannings and Thompson (1981, chap. 5). The series of genetic studies that provided the data for the example of section 3.6 are reviewed by Neel (1978), and many further references are given in that paper. While the theory of Dempster, Laird, and Rubin (1977) undoubtedly has applications in pedigree analysis (Smith 1957; Thompson 1983a), the precise methodology of its application in the reconstruction of genealogies remains to be pursued.

4. Probabilities on Pedigrees

4.1. Reasons for requiring probabilities

Chapter 2 has shown that gene identity is the basis of similarity between relatives, and in principle section 2.6 provides a method for the computation of joint phenotype probabilities. However, the number of identity states is too large for this to be an effective approach to the general problem of the computation of probabilities on large and complex genealogies. This chapter will develop more practicable procedures, but first let us address the question, what is the purpose of such computations? In fact, every problem of genetic data on related individuals requires them, and problems may be classified by whichever of the three basic elements of the situation is the unknown. These elements are the genealogical structure itself, the mode of inheritance (genetic model) for the trait of interest, and the observable phenotypes of individuals (figure 20).

Estimation of the first of these elements has already been considered; that is, as shown in chapter 3, where traits of known mode of inheritance are observed, questions about the genealogical structure can be answered by considering the likelihood for any hypothesized genealogy. More precisely,

P(observed phenotypes | known inheritance model,
hypothesized genealogy)

is the required likelihood. Alternatively, the genealogical structure may already be known and a trait observed on some members of it. The natural questions are then about the mode of inheritance of this trait, for now

P(observed phenotypes | hypothesized genetic model,
known genealogy)

is the likelihood for the hypothesized mode of inheritance. The model may range from a simple comparison of dominant and recessive inheritance (section 1.3) or the estimation of allele frequencies for founder members of a population (sections 1.4, 5.3) to complex models involving unknown parameters of segregation or phenotypic expression and factors depending on the age, sex, or environment of individuals. Clearly, some classification of models and their parameters is required in order for comparable alternatives to be considered. A basic characterization of models is given in section 4.6, and more complex models are discussed in chapter 6. This text will not explore the more complex features of models used in genetic epidemiol-

Figure 20. The three perspectives of pedigree analysis

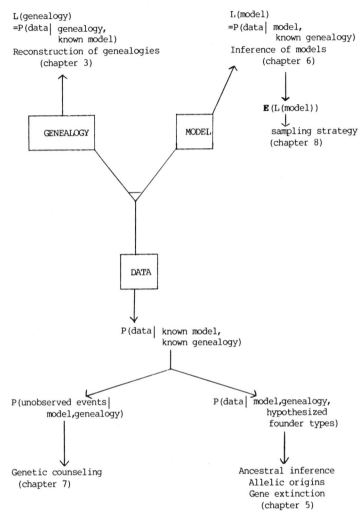

ogy, for little is known of the statistical behavior of likelihoods for such models on large and complex genealogies. Chapters 6 and 7 will, however, examine two practical examples of the fitting of simple models where the extended genealogy is necessary to the success of these particular studies.

The third area of pedigree analysis problems arises when both the genealogical structure and the modes of inheritance of traits are known. Then probabilities of phenotypic observations can be computed. The overall probability of observable phenotypes is unlikely now to be of interest, but conditional probabilities may be computed as the ratio of two joint ones (appendix 1):

P(event 1 *given* event 2) $= P$(both events) $/ P$(event 2).

This conditioning is used in computations of the probabilities of unobservable genotypes or phenotypes conditional on phenotypic observations made (figure 20). These are the classic genetic counseling questions. In most counseling situations, where perhaps the phenotypes of potential offspring of a single couple are in question, information on an extensive genealogy will be of little use. But where a trait is segregating in a large and complex genealogy, which perhaps constitutes the whole of an isolated population, it may be important to determine the joint distribution of current carriers of a recessive allele (chapter 7). In such cases it may also be of interest to trace the ancestral paths of such alleles, and this third area of pedigree analysis includes questions not only about the unobservable phenotypes of individuals who are not yet born, but also about the unobservable phenotypes and genotypes of those who are long since dead. Now,

P(observed phenotypes | known genetic model, known genealogy,
hypothesized founder genotypes)

is the likelihood for those hypothesized ancestral types. Questions about the types of the genes carried by the original founders of a population, or the origins of particular alleles, may be considered. Such questions are considered in chapter 5, where questions of gene extinction and survival also are discussed. These turn out to be closely related to questions of ancestry (section 4.8). Problems of the distributions of numbers of distinct genes surviving in isolated populations, and of the effects of genealogical structure on this distribution, thus also fall within the framework of pedigree analysis.

For any or all of these reasons the probability of given phenotypes on a given genealogy under a given genetic model must be computed. The remainder of this chapter will describe various methods for so doing, the different approaches being useful for different types of genealogy or genetic model. The next section outlines a method which is not normally of practical use, but which illustrates the general principles involved in such computations and introduces the form taken by probabilities on pedigrees.

4.2. Enumeration methods

Consider the small genealogy of figure 21 and a dominant trait determined by alleles at a single autosomal locus, the population frequency of the allele, a_1, for the trait being p, and $q = 1 - p$. Thus, this model is fully specified by the Hardy-Weinberg population frequencies of genotypes (section 1.4), the Mendelian segregation from parents to offspring (section 1.1), and the zero-one penetrances of the trait (section 1.3). The model is

Figure 21. An example genealogy for phenotype probability computation. A horizontal bar denotes an affected individual and a vertical bar denotes one known to be unaffected.

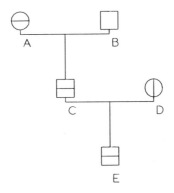

summarized in table 20. Suppose that individuals A, C, and E have the trait, D does not, and nothing is specified about individual B; the probability of this joint event is required. One way to determine this probability is to write down all genotype combinations for the individuals, the joint probability of each, and the conditional probability of phenotypes corresponding to each combination (table 21). Summing these contributions gives

$$pq^2(p^3 + p^2q + p^2q / 2 + pq^2 / 2 + p^2q + p^2q / 2 + pq^2$$
$$+ pq^2 + q^3 / 2)$$
$$= pq^2(p^3 + 3p^2q + 5pq^2 / 2 + q^3 / 2)$$
$$= (1/2)pq^2(2 - q^2) \qquad (26)$$

Of the total, $3^5 = 32$ potential genotype combinations, only the 9 of table 21 have nonzero probability and in this case the procedure is feasible. It would clearly not be so on a large genealogy.

Note the form of each contribution to the total probability. It involves the "population" probabilities for the genotypes of founders A, B, and D of the genealogy, multiplied, for A and D, by the relevant probability of phenotype given genotype ("penetrances"). Then there are also the relevant segregation ("transition") probabilities for nonfounders C and E, and their penetrance probabilities. The general form of any probability on any genealogy is thus

$$\Sigma_{\substack{\text{genotype} \\ \text{combinations}}} \quad [\{ \Pi_{\text{founders}} P(\text{genotype}) \}$$

$$\cdot \{ \Pi_{\text{nonfounders}} P(\text{genotype} \mid \text{parental genotype}) \}$$

$$\cdot \{ \Pi_{\substack{\text{observed} \\ \text{individuals}}} P(\text{phenotype} \mid \text{genotype}) \}],$$

Table 20. Model specification for a simple Mendelian dominant autosomal trait

Genotype i	a_1a_1	a_1a_2	a_2a_2
Population probability	p^2	$2pq$	q^2
Penetrances: P (affected $\mid i$)	1	1	0
P (normal $\mid i$)	0	0	1
Transitions:			
P (offspring $= i \mid$ parents)			
Parents $= a_1a_1, a_1a_1$	1	0	0
a_1a_1, a_1a_2	$1/2$	$1/2$	0
a_1a_2, a_1a_2	$1/4$	$1/2$	$1/4$
a_1a_1, a_2a_2	0	1	0
a_1a_2, a_2a_2	0	$1/2$	$1/2$
a_2a_2, a_2a_2	0	0	1

Table 21. Computation of a joint phenotype probability on the genealogy of figure 21

Individual genotypes of					Population probabilities			Penetrances		Segregations		Penetrances	
A	B	C	D	E	A	B	D	A	D	C	E	C	E
a_1a_1	a_1a_1	a_1a_1	a_2a_2	a_1a_2	p^2	p^2	q^2	1	1	1	1	1	1
a_1a_1	a_1a_2	a_1a_1	a_2a_2	a_1a_2	p^2	$2pq$	q^2	1	1	$1/2$	1	1	1
a_1a_1	a_1a_2	a_1a_2	a_2a_2	a_1a_2	p^2	$2pq$	q^2	1	1	$1/2$	$1/2$	1	1
a_1a_1	a_2a_2	a_1a_2	a_2a_2	a_1a_2	p^2	q^2	q^2	1	1	1	$1/2$	1	1
a_1a_2	a_1a_1	a_1a_1	a_2a_2	a_1a_2	$2pq$	p^2	q^2	1	1	$1/2$	1	1	1
a_1a_2	a_1a_1	a_1a_2	a_2a_2	a_1a_2	$2pq$	p^2	q^2	1	1	$1/2$	$1/2$	1	1
a_1a_2	a_1a_2	a_1a_1	a_2a_2	a_1a_2	$2pq$	$2pq$	q^2	1	1	$1/4$	1	1	1
a_1a_2	a_1a_2	a_1a_2	a_2a_2	a_1a_2	$2pq$	$2pq$	q^2	1	1	$1/2$	$1/2$	1	1
a_1a_2	a_2a_2	a_1a_2	a_2a_2	a_1a_2	$2pq$	q^2	q^2	1	1	$1/2$	$1/2$	1	1

Note: Total probability

$$= pq^2(p^3 + p^2q + 1/2\,p^2q + 1/2\,pq^2 + p^2q$$
$$+ 1/2\,p^2q + pq^2 + pq^2 + 1/2q^3)$$
$$= pq^2(p^3 + 3\,p^2q + 2 1/2\,pq^2 + 1/2q^3)$$
$$= pq^2(1 - 1/2\,pq^2 - 1/2q^3) = pq^2(1 - 1/2q^2).$$

Note also that the factors contributed by E depend on the genotypes of C and D, not on those of A and B.

where observed individuals are those whose phenotypes are specified. The problem is to find easier ways of computing and studying the behavior of this function. One small point to be noted is that the final product may be extended to cover all individuals by regarding the penetrance for an unspecified phenotype to be one regardless of genotype (table 20). In the example, B is the only individual without specified phenotype.

4.3. Recursive computation

Before proceeding to methods for computing probabilities on large genealogies, where there may be very large numbers of possible joint genotype combinations, a particular problem of descent probabilities will be considered. This problem can be solved by a recursive method. Denote by $g(A)$ the probability that a randomly chosen gene from an individual A derives by descent from one of a specified set of ancestral genes S in founders of the genealogy. Then, if M and F are the parents of A,

$$g(A) = (1/2)[g(M) + g(F)],$$

for the gene of A derives from M with probability $1/2$ and from F with probability $1/2$. If A is himself a founder, $g(A) = 0, 1/2,$ or 1 as $0, 1,$ or 2 genes of A are specified to be in the ancestral set S. This idea can be extended to more genes; let $g(A, B)$ denote the probability that genes chosen from each of A and B descend from some (either the same or different) gene(s) in S. Then, if A is not B nor an ancestor of B,

$$g(A, B) = (1/2) [g(M, B) + g(F, B)] \tag{27}$$

since again the maternal and paternal genes of A are each selected with probability $1/2$. Also,

$$g(A, A) = (1/2)[g(A) + g(M, F)], \tag{28}$$

for the two genes chosen successively from A either are the same gene twice over [probability $1/2$], this gene deriving from S with probability $g(A)$, or comprise both the maternal and paternal gene of A, also with probability $1/2$. For a founder A,

$$g(A, B) = 0, (1/2)g(B), \text{ or } g(B),$$

and

$$g(A, A) = 0, (1/4), \text{ or } 1, \text{ respectively,}$$

as

$0, 1,$ or 2 genes of A are in the ancestral set S.

Now note that equations (27) and (28) are precisely analogous to equations (9) and (10) of section 2.3, and can be implemented recursively in precisely the same way. Descent probabilities take a form that is very similar to kinship coefficients. As in that case, all probabilities will be of the form $r / 2^k$ for integers r and k, and may be computed exactly in this form. Using that same example genealogy (figure 6), suppose the following required probability: that two genes, one chosen randomly from D ($= 17$) and one from A ($= 13$), both descend from a given set of founder genes S. Suppose further that S consists of four genes, the maternal gene of 1, both genes of 2, and the paternal gene of 9. Then, as figure 22 shows, the recursive implementation of (27) and (28) is precisely analogous to figure 10, where the kinship coefficient $\psi(13, 17)$ was computed. The only difference is in the boundary conditions, where founders are encountered. Overall, the required probability is found to be $47/2^{10}$ (figure 22). As for the generalization of kinship coefficients to the multiple kinship coefficients of Karigl (1981), these equations also can be extended to consider the joint descent of larger numbers of genes (Thompson 1983c).

Why should these descent probabilities be of practical importance? Consider the genealogy of an isolated population descended from few founders. One problem often of interest in such populations is the segregation of recessive traits associated with medical conditions; such traits, normally rare, may attain substantial frequencies by repeated intermarriage of relatives. Suppose an individual A with parents M and F is affected by such a rare recessive trait. Then he must receive both his genes from the set of founder copies of the relevant allele. Let S denote a hypothesized set of such founder copies; then, if the hypothesis is correct, $g(M, F)$ is the probability that A is affected. Those sets S giving higher probability to the observed event that A is affected are, by definition, the more likely sets of ancestral copies, on the basis of this single data event. By comparing these bilateral descent probabilities $g(M, F)$ for alternative sets of hypothesized original copies of the allele, the likely such sets can be determined. Further, by considering descent jointly to both parents of A from sets of ancestral genes lower down the genealogy, the same method makes it possible to trace the likely paths of descent. Of course, one will normally wish to consider more a single individual A, and relationships between individuals of interest may make it necessary to consider the joint descent of larger numbers of genes, but the principle remains the same. An example is considered in the following section.

4.4. The origins of an allele in a Mennonite-Amish genealogy

The incidence of *propionic acidemia* in a large Mennonite-Amish genealogy is described by Kidd et al. (1980). This rare recessive disorder occurs in four current sibships, denoted A, B, C, and D (figure 23). It is possible for individuals to be affected (that is, to have the homozygous recessive genotype) without clinical symptoms, so phenotypes of unexam-

Figure 22. Recursive computation of descent probabilities. The four genes in the specified ancestral set S are the maternal gene of individual 1 (1_m), both genes of individual 2 (2_m, 2_p), and the paternal gene of individual 9 (9_p). The total probability that a gene chosen from each of 13 and 17 descends from this set is

$$3(1 + 1/2)2^{-8} + (1/4)2^{-5} + (1 + 1/2 + 1/2 + 1/4)2^{-8}$$
$$+ (1 + 1/2)2^{-7} = 47/2^{10}.$$

See figure 10 for a comparison with kinship computation.

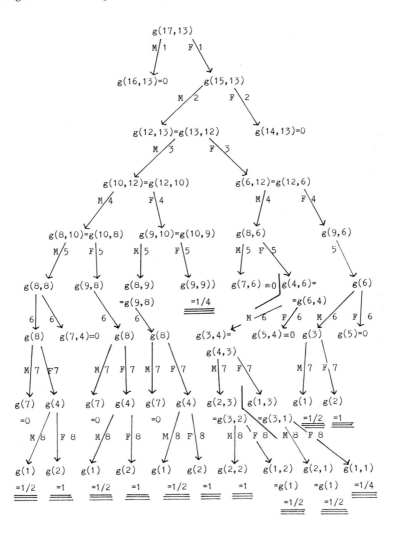

Figure 23. An outline of the Mennonite-Amish genealogy discussed in the text. Reprinted from Thompson 1983*b*. The outline shows original founders, and current sibships with affected individuals. In generation III, only the numbers of offspring ancestral to any affected sibship are given, and in generation XI only a representative affected individual is included. Each member of generation II is ancestral to every member of generation X, except II.5, who is an ancestor only of X.6. The close relationships between sibships *A*, *B*, and *C* are shown. The parents of sibship *D* are second cousins, but are not closely related to the other sibship parents. The full genealogy is given by Kidd et al. 1980.

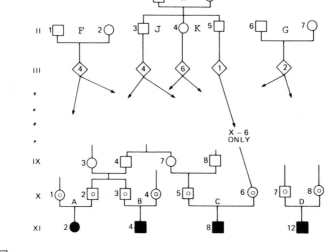

☐ male ancestor; phenotype unknown

◯ female ancestor; phenotype unknown

●■ representative of sibship containing one or more affected individuals

◇ sibship of 3 individuals, each ancestral to some individual of generation X

☐ ◉ parents of affected sibships; observed phenotypically normal

ined current individuals and of ancestors are not known with certainty, although it is likely that the majority are normal. The four sibships have been traced back to three couples, ten or eleven generations ago, each couple being ancestral to both the mother, *M*, and father, *F*, of each of the four sibships; so far as can be ascertained, these are the only such couples. These couples are denoted *E*, *F*, and *G*; they may well have been related, since the six individuals have, at most, four distinct surnames among them. The genealogy and data set thus constructed is biased, in that it considers only ancestry of known affected sibships. Nonetheless, it is of interest to consider the relative probabilities of descent to the four sibships from the "founder" couples, and/or from other ancestors. The extreme complexity of the genealogy over eleven generations makes other methods of computation very difficult, but the general form, with long chains of descent and large loops due to marriages between distant cousins, is ideal for recursive computation.

Each affected individual must have two copies of the allele—a_1, say—for propionic acidemia, and table 22 shows descent probabilities $g(M, F)$ for each pair of parents, M and F, of each of the four sibships. These descent probabilities are computed for a variety of ancestral sets of genes from the couples E, F, and G and provide relative likelihoods for the ancestral origin on the basis of each separate sibship containing affected individuals. Note that, as should be expected, descent probabilities increase as the set of ancestral genes is augmented. All founder genes being of type a_1 would give maximum probability of 1 to the event that any given current individual is affected, although this would be a rather implausible hypothesis. More precisely, since only descent of "affected genes" is considered, and not descent to the many normal individuals of the current population, the likelihood (based on these biased data) will favor more original genes of type a_1. Hypotheses of different numbers of ancestral genes are not strictly comparable, and for similar reasons care must be taken in comparing sets S at very different points in history. Nonetheless, it can be concluded that two of the sibships favor an allelic origin in couple E, and two in couple F, while the combination is as favored by all four sibships as any comparable alternative. Further, while the addition of couple G to couple E or couple F brings substantially increased descent probabilities, if both E and F are already assumed to carry the allele, the effect is smaller. In addition to E, F or G is likely to have carried the allele, but there is no strong reason to suppose that it is present in all three couples. The known shared surnames are in fact between E and F, and between F and G. Two of the offspring of couple E—J and K, say—also are ancestral to all eight sibship parents. One of these, J, is an important contributor, regardless of other hypotheses. The other makes a significant difference to the likelihoods only if F and G are *not* also carriers. However, on proceeding to the grandchildren of couple E, four are clearly implicated, these being two offspring of J and two of K. (In all, four offspring of J and six of K are ancestors of some affected individual.) This finding suggests that perhaps both J and K were carriers, in which case there is less support for the hypothesis that either couple F or couple G carried the allele.

All four of the affected sibships have closer interrelationships than obtain via the original couples. Indeed, the fathers of sibships A and B are brothers, and are cousins to the father of sibship C (figure 23). In inferring the likely origins of the a_1 allele, relative likelihoods cannot simply be combined over the four sibships. Instead, joint descent to all four sibships should be considered, but the recursive computation of descent probabilities is not readily extended to more than four genes (section 2.5). Table 23 gives some descent probabilities from a variety of ancestral sets simultaneously to sets of four parental genes. To show the degree of interaction in

Table 22. Exact probabilities $g(M, F) \times 2^{19}$ for the four sibships and for different ancestral sets

Ancestral set		Probability for sibship			
		A	B	C	D
One gene of couple	E	135	267	180	176
	F	180	200	24	220
	G	24	16	32	48
One gene in each of the couples	E, F	502	731	318	534
	F, G	280	280	136	376
	E, G	232	349	330	330
One gene in each of three couples	E, F, G	675	877	548	796

Table 23. Joint descent probabilities $\times 2^{36}$ for sets of four parent genes, and the ratio to the product of separate descent probabilities

	Ancestral set			
	One gene of E		One gene of E and F	
Current genes	Prob. $\times 2^{36}$	Ratio	Prob. $\times 2^{36}$	Ratio
A_m, B_m, C_m, D_m	7,873	16.7	60,979	4.9
A_m, B_m, C_m, D_p	31,482	42.8	149,418	9.6
A_m, B_m, C_p, D_m	9,667	18.7	107,299	5.7
A_m, B_m, C_p, D_p	31,032	38.5	246,741	10.6
A_m, B_p, C_m, D_m	9,363	7.5	61,478	3.7
A_m, B_p, C_m, D_p	35,938	43.5	134,580	6.5
A_m, B_p, C_p, D_m	27,126	29.9	185,506	7.5
A_m, B_p, C_p, D_p	79,034	56.0	366,550	11.9
A_p, B_m, C_m, D_m	21,081	10.6	95,595	3.9
A_p, B_m, C_m, D_p	66,642	21.6	208,916	6.9
A_p, B_m, C_p, D_m	64,714	29.7	305,427	8.3
A_p, B_m, C_p, D_p	152,516	45.1	599,344	13.2
A_p, B_p, C_m, D_m	153,228	44.1	503,900	15.6
A_p, B_p, C_m, D_p	444,660	82.3	935,944	23.4
A_p, B_p, C_p, D_m	498,616	130.9	1,770,032	36.5
A_p, B_p, C_p, D_p	1,090,476	184.1	2,798,004	46.6

Note: A_m denotes a maternal gene of sibship A; A_p, a paternal gene of that sibship.

Table 24. Probabilities $q(M, F) \times 2^{17}$ (to the nearest integer) of two heterozygous parents for each of the sibships and for various ancestral sets

		Sibship			
Ancestral set		A	B	C	D
One gene of couple	E	126	250	169	164
	F	172	190	24	207
	G	24	16	31	46
One gene in each of the couples	E, F	460	663	297	485
	F, G	267	266	131	349
	E, G	218	326	305	304
One gene in each of three couples	E, F, G	619	794	503	714

the descent lines, the ratios of these joint probabilities to the product of the four component descent probabilities also are given. Were the lines of descent independent, this product would be the joint probability (appendix 1). Table 23 shows the close relationships between the paternal genes of A, B, and C, and the four-parent descent probabilities also in fact confirm the previous conclusions as to likely allelic origins. However, the table also shows that combined relative likelihoods can differ substantially from those given by the separate sibships, and that there are strong effects of more remote relationships in interactions between sibships.

   In fact, more data are available than are included in the above computations. The eight parents of the four sibships were examined biochemically and were found to be phenotypically normal. Each must therefore carry precisely one copy of the a_1 allele, and for each pair of sibship parents the required descent probability is strictly not $g(M, F)$ but $q(M, F)$, (that is, in each of the parents precisely one gene descends from the ancestral set S). These probabilities can be determined from descent probabilities, but to arrive at them it is again necessary to consider sets of four genes (the four genes of each M and F pair). Equations are given by Thompson (1983b) but will not be pursued here, for provided the probability that M or F receives two genes from S is small compared to the probability of the one-gene event,

$g(M, F)$ is approximately $q(M, F) / 4$,

since if M and F do each have one gene from S, the probability that these are then chosen in randomly selecting a gene from each is $1/4$. Table 24 shows some probabilities $q(M, F)$. For easy comparison with table 22 these are given to the nearest integer multiple of 2^{17}, but the results are not exact.

The powers of $1/2$ actually involved are similar to those of table 23. Although somewhat smaller than the corresponding $4g(M, F)$ of table 22, the relative values are similar, and do not alter the previous inferences about the ancestral origins of the a_1 allele. Differences become greater as larger sets of genes are considered, for the probabilities that a parent M or F carries two genes descended from S are then increased. In other studies, knowledge that no such parent does so could alter inferences, and in general any available information on the types of both normal and affected individuals should be incorporated where computationally feasible.

4.5. Sequential computation

Return now to the example of section 4.2: there is an important feature of the contributions of table 21 that has not been commented upon. The two alternative genotypes of C partition the possibilities; the genotypes of A and B affect those of E only via that of C. For a given genotype of C, the three phenotype sets jointly of A and B, of C, and jointly of D and E are independent. This simple observation is the basis of methods providing probabilities on extended and complex genealogies for complicated genetic models. Individuals such as C, who divide a genealogy in this way, will be called *pivot* individuals.

Define

$$Q_X(i) = P(\text{data before } X \& X \text{ has genotype } i), \tag{29}$$

where the individuals are ordered as A, B, C, D, and E, and where "before" means strictly before in this ordering. As previously, "&" will be used to denote joint events whose intersection (appendix 1) is to be considered. Now,

$$Q_C(i) = P(\text{data on } A \text{ and } B \& \text{genotype of } C \text{ is } i)$$
$$= \Sigma_j \Sigma_k \, [P(\text{genotype } A \text{ is } k) \, P(\text{genotype } B \text{ is } j)$$
$$P(A \text{ affected} \mid \text{genotype } k)$$
$$P(\text{genotype } C \text{ is } i \mid \text{parents } j, k)]$$

(note that the phenotype of B is not specified), and

$$= \begin{cases} p^2 \cdot p^2 \cdot 1 \cdot 1 + p^2 \cdot 2pq \cdot (1/2) \cdot 1 + p^2 \cdot q^2 \cdot 0 \cdot 1 \\ + 2pq \cdot p^2 \cdot (1/2) \cdot 1 + 2pq \cdot 2pq \cdot (1/4) \cdot 1 \\ \qquad\qquad + 2pq \cdot q^2 \cdot 0 \cdot 1 \\ + q^2 \cdot p^2 \cdot 1 \cdot 0 + q^2 \cdot 2pq \cdot (1/2) \cdot 0 + q^2 \cdot q^2 \cdot 0 \cdot 0 \end{cases} \begin{array}{l} \text{for} \\ i = a_1 a_1 \end{array}$$

$$= \begin{cases} p^2 \cdot p^2 \cdot 0 \cdot 1 + p^2 \cdot 2pq \cdot (1/2) \cdot 1 + p^2 \cdot q^2 \cdot 1 \cdot 1 \\ + 2pq \cdot p^2 \cdot (1/2) \cdot 1 + 2pq \cdot 2pq \cdot (1/2) \cdot 1 \\ \qquad\qquad + 2pq \cdot q^2 \cdot (1/2) \cdot 1 \\ + q^2 \cdot p^2 \cdot 1 \cdot 0 + q^2 \cdot 2pq \cdot (1/2) \cdot 0 + q^2 \cdot q^2 \cdot 0 \cdot 0 \end{cases} \begin{array}{l} \text{for} \\ i = a_1 a_2 \end{array}$$

$$
= \left\{
\begin{array}{l}
p^2 \cdot p^2 \cdot 0 \cdot 1 + p^2 \cdot 2pq \cdot 0 \cdot 1 + p^2 \cdot q^2 \cdot 0 \cdot 1 \\
+ 2pq \cdot p^2 \cdot 0 \cdot 1 + 2pq \cdot 2pq \cdot (1/4) \cdot 1 \\
\qquad + 2pq \cdot q^2 \cdot (1/2) \cdot 1 \\
+ q^2 \cdot p^2 \cdot 0 \cdot 0 + q^2 \cdot 2pq \cdot (1/2) \cdot + q^2 \cdot q^2 \cdot 1 \cdot 0
\end{array}
\right\}
\begin{array}{l}
\text{for} \\
i = a_2 a_2
\end{array}
$$

$$
\left\{
\begin{array}{ll}
= p^2(p^2 + pq + pq + q^2) = p^2 & \text{for } i = a_1 a_1 \\
= pq(p^2 + pq + p^2 + 2pq + q^2) = pq(p + 1) & \text{for } i = a_1 a_2 \\
= pq^2(p + q) = pq^2 & \text{for } i = a_2 a_2.
\end{array}
\right.
$$

In this one case all nine terms of each summation are included. In the future, terms that are clearly zero, due either to the segregation factor or to the specified phenotype, will be omitted. In fact, since C is to be affected he cannot be $a_2 a_2$, and the third term, $Q_C(a_2 a_2)$, above is irrelevant.

Now proceed to the family C, D, E;

$$
\begin{aligned}
Q_E(i) &= P(\text{data before } E \& E \text{ has genotype } i) \\
&= \Sigma_j [P(\text{data before } C \& C \text{ has genotype } j) \, P(C \text{ affected} \mid \text{genotype } j) \\
&\qquad \Sigma_k [P(D \text{ has genotype } k) \, P(D \text{ normal} \mid \text{genotype } k) \\
&\qquad\qquad P(E \text{ has genotype } i \mid \text{parents } j, k)]
\end{aligned}
$$

$$
\left\{
\begin{array}{ll}
= Q_C(a_1 a_1) \cdot q^2 \cdot 0 + Q_C(a_1 a_2) \cdot q^2 \cdot 0 & \text{for } i = a_1 a_1 \\
= Q_C(a_1 a_1) \cdot q^2 \cdot 1 + Q_C(a_1 a_2) \cdot q^2 \cdot (1/2) & \text{for } i = a_1 a_2 \\
= Q_C(a_1 a_1) \cdot q^2 \cdot 0 + Q_C(a_1 a_2) \cdot q^2 \cdot (1/2) & \text{for } i = a_2 a_2
\end{array}
\right.
$$

$$
\left\{
\begin{array}{ll}
= 0 & \text{for } i = a_1 a_1 \\
= q^2 p^2 + (1/2)pq^3(p + 1) & \text{for } i = a_1 a_2 \\
= (1/2) \, pq^3(p + 1) & \text{for } i = a_2 a_2.
\end{array}
\right.
$$

Again, although included for generality of the procedure, the final term, $Q_E(a_2 a_2)$, will prove to be irrelevant. For the total overall probability is

$$
\begin{aligned}
&\Sigma_i [P(\text{data before } E \& E \text{ has genotype } i) \cdot P(E \text{ affected} \mid \text{genotype } i)] \\
&= Q_E(a_1 a_1) \cdot 1 + Q_E(a_1 a_2) \cdot 1 + Q_E(a_2 a_2) \cdot 0 \\
&= q^2 p^2 + (1/2)p^2 q^3 + (1/2)pq^3 \\
&= (1/2)pq^2(2p + pq + q) = (1/2)pq^2(2 - q^2),
\end{aligned}
$$

which is the same result as that obtained in equation (26).

Although it is genetically more intuitive to regard D and E as independent of A and B given the genotype of C, probabilistically the reverse is equally true. Information on the phenotypes of D and E jointly affects probabilities for the genotype of C, but only thence affects those for A and B. Thus, it is possible to work up genealogies as well as down them, combining first the information from D and E onto the pivot C. However, to do so it is necessary to work with slightly different probability functions;

$$
L_X(i) = P(\text{data after } X \mid X \text{ has genotype } i), \tag{30}
$$

where, as for "before" above, "after" means strictly after in the ordering A, B, C, D, E. These conditional probabilities are denoted L since they are *likelihoods* for the genotype of X, given only the genetic data on individuals following him in the ordering. This interpretation of these probabilities will be used to address the problem of ancestral origins of alleles in chapter 5. However, unless that interpretation is found helpful, understanding it may be deferred for the present. Here the functions L_X are manipulated purely as the conditional probabilities of events. These probabilities, L_X, obey equations that are very similar to those for Q_X above. Given the genotype of C, the probability of data on D and E is

$$L_C(i) = \Sigma_j\{ P(\text{genotype of } D \text{ is } j) \, P(D \text{ is normal} \mid \text{genotype } j)$$
$$\Sigma_k[P(\text{genotype of } E \text{ is } k \mid \text{parents } i,j)$$
$$P(E \text{ is affected} \mid \text{genotype } k)]\}$$

$$\begin{cases} = q^2(0 \cdot 1 + 1 \cdot 1 + 0 \cdot 0) & \text{for } i = a_1a_1 \\ = q^2[0 \cdot 1 + (1/2) \cdot 1 + (1/2) \cdot 0] & \text{for } i = a_1a_2 \\ = q^2(0 \cdot 1 + 0 \cdot 1 + 1 \cdot 0) & \text{for } i = a_2a_2. \end{cases}$$

Now all information from D and E is summarized into the contributions $L_C(i)$, and the same form of recurrence equation can be applied to the family A, B, C;

$$L_A(i) = \Sigma_j\{ P(\text{genotype of } B \text{ is } j)$$
$$\Sigma_k[P(\text{genotype of } C \text{ is } k \mid \text{parents } i,j)$$
$$P(C \text{ is affected} \mid \text{genotype } k)$$
$$P(\text{data after } C \mid C \text{ has genotype } k)]\}$$

$$\begin{cases} = q^2[p^2 \cdot 1 + 2pq \cdot (1/2 + 1/4) + q^2 \cdot (1/2)] & \text{for } i = a_1a_1 \\ = q^2[p^2 \cdot (1/2 + 1/4) + 2pq \cdot (1/4 + 1/4) \\ \quad + q^2 \cdot (1/4)] & \text{for } i = a_1a_2 \\ = q^2[p^2 \cdot (1/2) + 2pq \cdot (1/4)] & \text{for } i = a_2a_2 \end{cases}$$

Finally, the overall probability is

$$\Sigma_i[P(\text{genotype of } A \text{ is } i)P(A \text{ is affected} \mid \text{genotype } i)$$
$$P(\text{data after } A \mid A \text{ has genotype } i)]$$
$$= p^2 \cdot 1 \cdot L_A(a_1a_1) + 2pq \cdot 1 \cdot L_A(a_1a_2) + q^2 \cdot 0 \cdot L_A(a_2a_2),$$

which again reduces to $(1/2) \, pq^2(2 - q^2)$. Thus, it is possible to work up a genealogy; at each stage the contributions from individuals after X in the genealogy are combined into the three terms of $L_X(i)$ for each pivot individual X in turn.

4.6. Components of a model, and computations on genealogies without loops

The method of the above section does not, for this example, seem simpler than the enumeration of table 21. Its advantage is that it can be generalized to far more complex problems without increasing the difficulty of the computation. Consider first the generalization of the genetic model. In the description of table 20, which provides all the components required to determine the probability, three factors are specified:

"Population": $R(j) = P$(random member of the population has genotype j)

"Penetrances": $S_A(j) = P(A$ has phenotype specified | genotype of A is j)

"Transition": $T(i \mid j, k) = P$(child has genotype i | parents j, k)

This specification of models was introduced by Elston and Stewart (1971) and covers wide classes of traits. One requirement is that S must summarize the genotype/phenotype relationship; phenotypes of relatives are correlated only via their genotypes. But the penetrance functions need not take only values zero or one, and can depend on the age, sex, or environment of the individual. Another requirement is that the transition of genotype must be summarized by T; offspring are conditionally independent given genotypes of parents (OCIGGOP models). But T is not restricted to Mendelian segregation at autosomal loci. T may describe the segregation of genes at X-linked loci (section 1.3) or at several linked loci (1.6), or even the segregation of polygenic effects (1.7). In addition, the possibility of segregation distortion (non-50:50 segregation in heterozygotes) is clearly covered. Finally, population frequencies must be specifiable by $R(j)$ independently for each founder individual, but in fact, as section 6.4 will show, dependence between spouses (hence assortative mating) can be incorporated. Even for the case of independent founders the frequencies $R(j)$ need not be the standard $(p^2, 2pq, q^2)$, although for the sake of simplicity this is the most frequently used form. There may be deviations from Hardy-Weinberg frequencies, or $R(j)$ could denote the population frequencies of polygenic values (section 6.2).

Now, for example, the first two sets of equations of the previous section become

$$Q_C(i) = \Sigma_j \Sigma_k [R(j) \ R(k) \ S_A(k) \ T(i \mid j, k)]$$

and

$$Q_E(i) = \Sigma_j \{ Q_C(j) \ S_C(j) \ \Sigma_k [R(k) \ S_D(k) \ T(i \mid j, k)] \} .$$

The other equations for Q and L all have similar forms, which the reader may want to determine to achieve familiarity with the notation.

Consider second the generalization of the genealogical form, first to all genealogies without loops. The point of the method is that computation on any such genealogy is no more difficult than on the two connected parent-offspring triplets of this example. Summation over a maximum of two sets of genotypes at any stage will prove sufficient, however large the genealogy. On large genealogies, of course, the computations are not done by hand. Yet, using these equations, the time required for computation increases only linearly with the size of the genealogy, and the number of items the computer must hold for future stages in the computation remains roughly constant. An essentially universal form of the equations of the previous section enables one to program the procedure easily.

In a genealogy without loops (figure 24), each person, B, divides the genealogy into three mutually exclusive and exhaustive (possibly empty) parts. One part consists of B himself, while the other two are the "before" and "after" parts previously considered. Since many different orderings of the individuals could be considered, these two parts will now be renamed "above" and "below," which can be defined unambiguously. The individuals *above B* are those connected to him via his parents, including his sibs, sibs' descendants, and these descendants' ancestors. (Note that the partition does not have chronological interpretation.) The individuals *below B* are those connected to him via his offspring, including his spouse(s) and their ancestors. Note that there can be several nonoverlapping subsets of "below" individuals if B has several spouses. Although this complication will not be considered explicitly, the reader should note that in the examples care must be taken to include contributions from all these subsections; also, that "above" and "below" are not reciprocal; 3 and 12 are below 1 in figure 24, while 1 is below 12 but above 3.

The definitions of Q and L now read

$Q_B(i) = P(\text{data above } B \,\&\, B \text{ has genotype } i)$ [see equation (29)];
$L_B(i) = P(\text{data below } B \mid B \text{ has genotype } i)$ [see equation (30)].

If there are no individuals above B, then

$Q_B(i) = P(B \text{ has genotype } i) = R(i).$

Figure 24. An example genealogy without loops

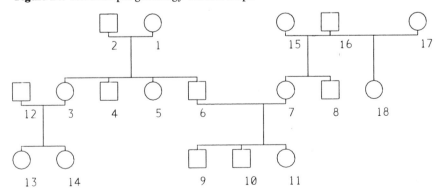

If there are no individuals below B, convention dictates

$L_B(i) = 1$.

Recall also that where the phenotype of an individual is not specified,

$S_B(i) = 1$ for each i.

With these conventions, the equations of section 4.5 take a single form. When working down the genealogy, from parents M and F to a single offspring B,

$$Q_B(i) = \Sigma_j \Sigma_k [Q_M(j) \, Q_F(k) \, S_M(j) \, S_F(k) \, T(i \,|\, j, k)]. \qquad (31)$$

When working up the genealogy, each offspring C contributes independently to the parental genotype combination (i, j) a factor

$$\Sigma_k [S_C(k) \, T(k \,|\, i, j) \, L_C(k)] = L_{M,F}^*(C : i, j), \text{ say.} \qquad (32)$$

It is now possible to work through any genealogy without loops. At any stage information can be accumulated from any family in which there remains only one individual connected to the core of the unanalyzed genealogy. The equations for the genealogy of figure 23 are given as an example. These are not the only possibilities; there are different orderings of families which allow the accumulation of contributions to give the same overall probability. Some orderings may be computationally more efficient than others, optimality depending mainly on the subset of individuals for which phenotypes are specified. The validity and form of the equations are, however, independent of knowledge of this subset.

Consider first the left-most family, and the contributions of phenotypic data (if any) on 13 and 14 to the genotype probabilities for their parents 12 and 3, adding these, and any information on 12, to an L function on the pivot 3:

$$L_{3,12}^*(13 : i, j) = \Sigma_k [L_{13}(k) \, T(k \,|\, i, j) \, S_{13}(k)],$$
$$L_{3,12}^*(14 : i, j) = \Sigma_k [L_{14}(k) \, T(k \,|\, i, j) \, S_{14}(k)],$$

where $L_{13}(k) = L_{14}(k) = 1$ for each k, since 13 and 14 have no descendants.

$$L_3(i) = \Sigma_j [Q_{12}(j) \, S_{12}(j) \, L_{3,12}^*(13 : i, j) \, L_{3,12}^*(14 : i, j)],$$

where $Q_{12}(j) = R(j)$, since there are no individuals above 12. In the above and following equations the factors for peripheral individuals are given in general form, allowing for the possibility that further families connect to them, and the fact is noted separately that $L(k) = 1$ or $Q(k) = R(k)$ if the genealogy is only as shown.

Now any information of 12, 13, and 14 has been accumulated into L_3, and now contributions from data on offspring 3, 4, and 5 to probabilities for their parents, 1 and 2, may likewise be accumulated:

$$L^*_{1,2}(3:i,j) = \Sigma_k[L_3(k)\ T(k\,|\,i,j)\ S_3(k)],$$

$L_3(k)$ having been computed;

$$L^*_{1,2}(4:i,j) = \Sigma_k[L_4(k)\ T(k\,|\,i,j)\ S_4(k)],$$

where $L_4(k) = 1$ for each k;

$$L^*_{1,2}(5:i,j) = \Sigma_k[L_5(k)\ T(k\,|\,i,j)\ S_5(k)],$$

where $L_5(k) = 1$ for each k.
Let

$$L^{**}_{1,2}(i,j) = L^*_{1,2}(3:i,j)\ L^*_{1,2}(4:i,j)\ L^*_{1,2}(5:i,j),$$

which contains information from all the offspring, and individuals below them, apart from offspring 6. Thus, the information may be accumulated onto individual 6, including also any phenotypic data on individuals 1 and 2:

$$Q_6(i) = \Sigma_j\Sigma_k[Q_1(j)\ Q_2(k)\ S_1(j)\ S_2(k)\ T(i\,|\,j,k)\ L^{**}_{1,2}(j,k)].$$

Similarly, for the next family

$$L^*_{6,7}(9:i,j) = \Sigma_k[L_9(k)\ T(k\,|\,i,j)\ S_9(k)],$$

where $L_9(k) = 1$ for each k, and similarly for offspring 10 and 11. Combining the contributions

$$L^{**}_{6,7}(i,j) = L^*_{6,7}(9:i,j)\ L^*_{6,7}(10:i,j)\ L^*_{6,7}(11:i,j),$$

accumulating all the information already combined into $Q_6(i)$, and incorporating any phenotypic information on 6,

$$L_7(j) = \Sigma_i[Q_6(i)\ S_6(i)\ L^{**}_{6,7}(i,j)].$$

Now, in addition, information on 7 is incorporated by

$$L^*_{15,16}(7:i,j) = \Sigma_k[L_7(k)\ T(k\,|\,i,j)\ S_7(k)],$$

while

$$L^*_{15,16}(8:i,j) = \Sigma_k[L_8(k)\ T(k\,|\,i,j)\ S_8(k)],$$

where $L_8(k) = 1$ for each k. Thus, for the subsection of individuals below 16 but corresponding only to spouse 15,

$$L_{16}(i) = \Sigma_j[Q_{15}(j)\ S_{15}(j)\ L^*_{15,16}(7:j,i)\ L^*_{15,16}(8:j,i)],$$

where $Q_{15}(j) = R(j)$. Then

$$Q_{18}(i) = \Sigma_j\Sigma_k[Q_{16}(k)\ L_{16}(k)\ Q_{17}(j)\ S_{16}(k)\ S_{17}(j)\ T(k\,|\,i,j)],$$

where $Q_{16}(k) = Q_{17}(k) = R(k)$ for each k, since 16 and 17 are founders. Finally, the total overall probability is

$\Sigma_i [Q_{18}(i) \; L_{18}(i) \; S_{18}(i)]$,

where $L_{18}(i) = 1$ for each i.

There is an important feature of the above equations. The functions Q and L have different meanings, and for interpretation of values must be carefully distinguished. But the equations for working up and working down a genealogy take the same form, with Q or L, or both, being inserted as appropriate. Thus, in programming the method, no distinction is made. The program need not specify whether one is progressing up or down a genealogy, but only which individuals are offspring, which are parents, and which is the pivot member of the family.

4.7. Computations on complex genealogies

It is not sufficient to be able to compute probabilities on genealogies without loops. Large genealogies of isolated populations will always include marriages between relatives, and couples in which each member of a pair is related to each member of another (for example, two sisters marrying two brothers). A small genealogy that illustrates several of the features of more complicated examples is shown in figure 25. The marriage node graph (section 2.2) of the same genealogy also is shown. The problem is that an individual—for example, 6—may no longer divide the genealogy; "above 6" and "below 6" are not mutually exclusive for 34 is both above 6 (via 8) and below 6 (via 33). Thus, a given genotype for 6 affects the genotype probability for 34 first via her brother 8. But even given a genotype for individual 8, if there are data on individual 31, individuals 6 and 34 will still be interdependent via resulting genotype probabilities on 31's parents 33 and 34 (33 being the child of 6). Further, even if a separate genotype is specified for 8 and for 33, data on 30 will still induce dependence in the joint genotype probabilities for 6 and 34, for 30 is the grandchild of 34 and the great-great-great-nephew (via 10) of 6. Only if they are conditioned upon genotypes for 33, 8, and 10 (or upon other equivalent sets) will 6 and 34 be independent. This situation can be visualized as these three individuals *cutting* all the links between 6 and 34.

Thus, a genealogy may be divided by *cutsets* of several individuals. For set $\{33, 8, 10\}$, for example, there is clearly an above and a below. Q and L functions may be defined for any such set;

$$Q_{33,8,10}(i, j, k) = P(\text{data above } \{33, 8, 10\} \; \& \; \text{genotype of 33 is } i \; \& \\ \text{genotype of 8 is } j \; \& \; \text{genotype of 10 is } k)$$

and

$$L_{33,8,10}(i, j, k) = P(\text{data below } \{33, 8, 10\} \mid \text{genotype of 33 is } i, \\ \text{of 8 is } j, \text{ and of 10 is } k).$$

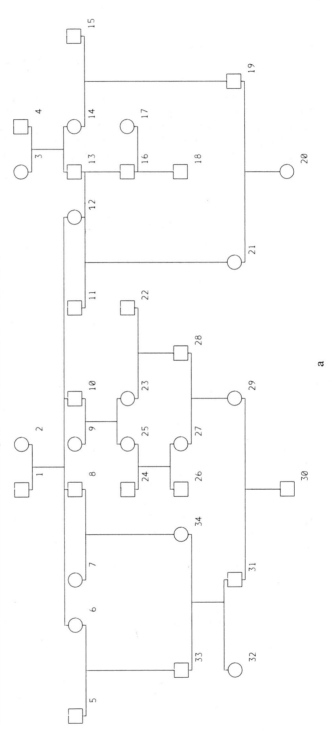

Figure 25. The genealogy for the complex example discussed in the text: (*a*) in classical form; (*b*) in marriage node graph form. In case (*b*) two cutsets are shown, one consisting of individuals 31, 25, and 23, the other of individuals 13 and 21.

a

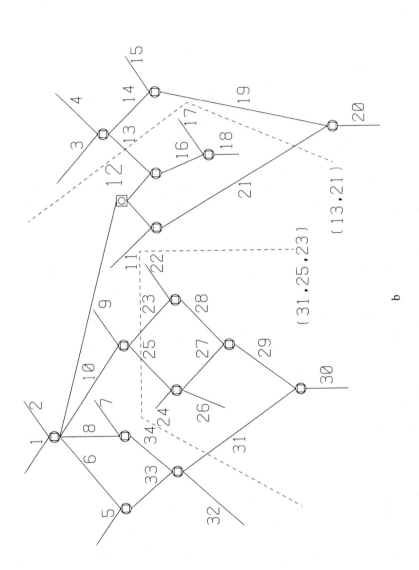

b

Set $\{31, 25, 23\}$ is another for which there is an above and a below. It would not divide 6 and 34, but, for example, for specified genotypes of 31, 25, and 23, data on 29, who is below the set, would be independent of that on 34, who is above. The genealogy is also divided by set $\{13, 21\}$, but the two sections are "above 13 and below 21," and vice versa. Fortunately, since the distinction between Q and L functions is not necessary in programming, this does not cause problems. A mixed "Q-L type" function may be defined:

$$P(\text{data above 13 \& below 21 \& genotype of 13 is } i \mid \text{genotype of 21 is } j).$$

With these joint functions over the genotype combinations for sets of individuals in *cutsets* dividing the genealogy, it is possible to work through a genealogy sequentially, in a manner very similar to the case of a genealogy without loops. Since the equations are cumbersome, and only the principle is important here, I will not describe this method in full. However, table 25 shows a sequence that would allow rapid computation on this genealogy.

If there are G genotypes, then any one of K individuals to be considered jointly has potentially G alternative types, and there are, in all, G^K combinations. This is therefore the number of terms in one of the above functions on a cutset of K individuals. This increases rapidly with K, and even for simple models ($G = 3$), restrictions on store make it impossible to consider sets of more than eight or nine individuals. However, this number does allow large and complicated genealogies to be considered; for the one in the above example the maximum K required is 3. It may also be possible to subdivide the problem, or first to restrict the number of individuals of unknown genotype by the use of phenotypic information. Also, while some possible orderings may give an unacceptably large maximum K, an alternative sequence may give a smaller one. For example, it would have been possible to use $\{33, 34, 27, 28\}$ as one of the sets in table 25, but since this requires $K = 4$, the sequence given there is preferable. The efficient determination of sequences minimizing the maximum K is an interesting unsolved problem. Although some results of graph theory apply, they tend not to provide practical answers. When working from one cutset to the next, the total number of distinct individuals in the two combined sets, K^*, is important. Analogous to the total given above, the potential total number of terms in all the transition equations here is G^{K^*}. Restriction on computation time requires that, normally, K^* be no more than 13 or 14 for $G = 3$. In some cases it may again be possible to restrict the combinations considered, by efficient elimination of zero contributions to the equations.

4.8. Ancestral likelihoods and extinction probabilities

Using the above methods, it is possible to compute joint probabilities of phenotypic data on a genealogy. By including specified founder types as

Table 25. Cutset sequence for the example of figure 25

Individuals in cutset	Additional individuals from whom data have been accumulated	Type of function	Number in cutset	Number in computation
First consider:				
13, 14	3, 4	Q	2	4
13, 19	14, 15	Q	2	4
13, 21	19, 20	$Q - L$	2	4
13, 12	11, 21	$Q - L$	2	4
A separate computation gives:				
16	17, 18	L	1	3
12, 13	16	L	2	3
Combining the above two sets gives:				
12	13	L	1	2
Starting a new computation, we have:				
31, 29	30	L	2	3
31, 27, 28	29	L	3	4
31, 25, 28	24, 26, 27	L	3	6
31, 25, 23	28, 22	L	3	5
31, 10	9, 25, 23	L	2	5
33, 34, 10	32, 31	L	3	5
6, 34, 10	5, 33	L	3	5
6, 8, 10	7, 34	L	3	5
1, 2	6, 8, 10	$L*$	2	5
12	1, 2	Q	1	3

Finally, combining the Q and L functions on 12 gives the overall probability $\Sigma_i \, Q_{12}(i) \, L_{12}(i) \, S_{12}(i)$.

Notes: The sequence of operations is fully described in the text. Maximum cutset = 3; $3^3 = 27$. Maximum number of individuals in the computation = 6; $3^6 = 729$.
*Only contributions via offspring 6, 8, and 10, and not 12, are included.

additional "data," it is also possible to compute the probabilities of current observations conditional upon the specified combination of founder genotypes. Suppose the genealogy were sufficiently small, and the founders sufficiently few, for us to work back through the genealogy toward a final cutset consisting of all the founders. Then the function finally computed would be (see section 4.1)

$$L_{\text{founders}} \text{(founder genotype set)} = P(\text{observed data} \mid \text{founder genotypes}),$$

that is, the set of probabilities of all observed phenotypic data conditional on each possible genotypic combination over these founders. With one computation, a likelihood function over all founder combinations could be obtained. Further, this likelihood would not depend upon any assumed allele frequencies; allele frequencies enter the computation only where downward probabilities Q are inserted for founders, and not where the computation is entirely in terms of L (conditional) probabilities.

Few genealogies of interest are sufficiently small for this method to be feasible. Yet there may be some small subgroup of founders of particular interest that could be taken as the final cutset. In this case some allele frequencies would have to be assumed, to provide the genotype probabilities of other founders, but subject to these assumed values, again one could obtain a complete set of probabilities of all observed phenotypic data conditional on each genotype combination in the founder set of interest. Of course, these likelihoods and relative likelihoods would vary with the allele frequencies assumed for other founders, and different computations would be required in order to consider a variety of allele frequencies for the founders not of interest. This approach will be pursued further in chapter 5.

Consider finally the problem of extinction of a specified set, S, of founder genes, in addition to the possible extinction of other genes. This can be solved by considering a hypothetical diallelic Mendelian autosomal locus. Label the genes of S as some allelic type—a_1, say—and all other founder genes as a_2. Then, at least the genes of S would be extinct if every member of the current population had genotype $a_2 a_2$. Thus, the probability of extinction of at least the genes of S is the probability of current genotypes $a_2 a_2$ conditional on the specified ancestral genotype combination—that is, an ancestral likelihood (figure 26). Conversely, from the "data" of $a_2 a_2$ individuals, and assuming also $a_2 a_2$ input from some founders, it is possible to work back to a complete ancestral likelihood function on the genotype combinations of the remaining subset of founders—that is, simultaneously, the set of extinction probabilities for every subset of the genes of this group of founders. This single computation suffices for any analysis of the joint survival or extinction of genes in any members of this group. Gene extinction will be considered briefly in chapter 5, for the particular example of the Tristan da Cunha population, but the main importance of this topic lies in theoretical studies of the effect of genealogical structure on the distributions of numbers of surviving genes. These are outside the scope of this text.

4.9. Further reading

The literature on use of computational methods on genealogies is extensive; not all the relevant papers can be cited. Earlier investigators em-

Figure 26. Extinction probabilities as ancestral likelihoods. The event of extinction of (at least) all the genes labeled a_1 in the founders is precisely the event that only a_2a_2 individuals exist in the current population, given the specified combination of founder genes. The extinction probability is thus the likelihood of the founder gene combination, given a current population of a_2a_2 individuals.

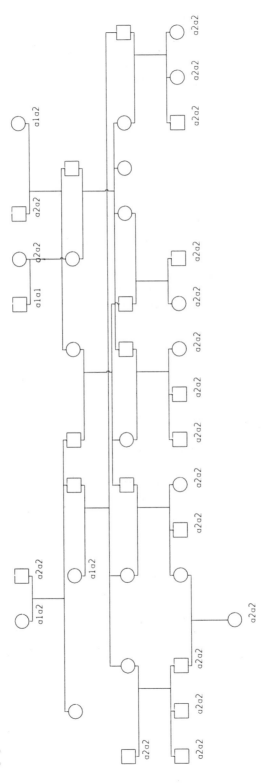

ployed enumerative methods, but these reached their limit with Ott (1974) and Cannings et al. (1976). By then, sequential methods were becoming more widely recognized, with Hilden (1970) giving a theoretical framework for, in principle, working down even complex genealogies, and Heuch and Li (1972) working both up and down genealogies without loops; but both of these studies used only very specific, simple genetic models. Elston and Stewart (1971) worked only up simple genealogies but generalized the framework of models under which this could be done. Smith (1976) gave a clear account of working both up and down small genealogies without loops, and Lange and Elston (1975) extended Elston and Stewart (1971) to more complex genealogies. Cannings, Thompson, and Skolnick (1978) completed this phase of development with the theory and procedures for working both up and down much more complicated genealogies with multiply interconnected loops. More recent developments have been in the area of applications to complex genetic models, and are discussed in chapter 6. Thompson (1976*d*, 1977) gives the programs and practical details of the procedures of Cannings, Thompson, and Skolnick (1978), while applications to problems of ancestral inference and gene extinction on the complex genealogies are discussed by Thompson, Cannings, and Skolnick (1978).

Although recursive methods have been known in principle for many years, and implemented by hand in some instances, they have become useful tools on large genealogies only with the advent of recursive, block-structured computer languages. Rostron (1978) gives a recursive computer algorithm for pairwise kinship coefficients, while Karigl (1981) generalizes the theory to larger numbers of genes. Thompson (1980*a*) includes some simple recursive routines for searching out and sorting genealogies, and for making simple computations thereon, while Thompson (1983*b*, 1983*c*) extends the ideas of Karigl (1981) to questions of ancestral origins of alleles. Kidd et al. (1980) give details of the study used in section 4.4 above as an example of recursive computation. It seems likely that recursive methods will solve more computational problems in the near future, but their use is limited to rather simple genetic models. Thus, sequential methods are unlikely to be superseded in the area of estimation and inference of genetic models, which will be described in chapter 6.

5. The Genes of the Tristan da Cunhans

5.1. The history of the population

Tristan da Cunha, a small island in the South Atlantic, was discovered in 1506 by a Portuguese admiral of that name. The island is a volcano roughly 7 miles in diameter, and only 3 of its 38 square miles are suitable for cultivation. The island lies 1,750 miles west of Cape Town, more than 2,000 miles east of Buenos Aires and 1,350 miles south of St. Helena, which is its center of local government. During the three centuries following its discovery, the island had a varied history of exploration and abortive attempts at settlement. However, its remoteness and its inhospitable climate and terrain counteracted its strategic attraction as a permanent base for merchant or naval shipping.

In 1815, at the Congress of Vienna, the island was annexed to Great Britain. In 1816 a garrison was sent to the island in the belief that this might deter any attempt to rescue the emperor Napoleon, who was then in exile on St. Helena! Some members of the garrison took their wives and children with them, and the first recorded birth on the island occurred later in that same year. However, in 1817 the garrison was withdrawn, the expense of maintaining it being deemed greater than its deterrent value. Three members of the garrison—one a corporal with a wife and children—asked if they could remain as settlers and were granted permission to do so. The two single men did not, in fact, remain long, but over the next ten years additional settlers came and went. By 1827 there were five male settlers in addition to the garrison corporal and his rapidly growing family. Recognizing that the current sex ratio was not conducive to a permanent settlement, the men asked the governor of St. Helena to send some women to the island. In due course, five arrived, and despite doubts (on all sides) as to their desirability and suitability, today three are represented by large numbers of descendants. These three were two sisters and the daughter of one of them, and so in terms of genetic contribution are more easily considered the parents of the sisters and the father of the daughter, although these three parent individuals were never on the island.

Soon after this rather unpropitious start, the population began to increase rapidly, and in 1852 the number of inhabitants of the thriving community first topped 100. In 1853, however, the original founder, the corporal, died, and many of his descendants, finding that they no longer enjoyed a privileged position in the community, left the island shortly afterward. By 1858 the population had decreased to 33, but the hard core remained, and thereafter the size of the community slowly increased again. This bottleneck was responsible for the small number of contributors to the current population. The total set of early founders consisted of the original Scots corporal and his wife, two Englishmen, two Americans, one Dutchman, and the three St. Helenans, who were probably half-negro. Together with another St. Helenan woman, who remained on the island after surviving a shipwreck in 1863 and today is represented by many descendants, this small but ethnically varied set of individuals contributed over 80 percent of the current population's genes. The marriage relationships of these individuals are shown in figure 27, and their origins and the number of their current descendants are given in table 26.

By the mid 1880s the population had again reached 100. The island was no longer an important landmark for shipping en route from Australia and the East Indies, however, and the community had suffered an economic decline. In 1885, disaster struck: 15 of the 16 nonsenile adult men were drowned when the islanders' boat went down. Many thought this would mean the end of the population, but again the islanders proved equal to the challenge. Some did leave, but a new fishing boat was donated and was in operation by 1886, manned by the community's teen-age boys. There were very few births on the island for several years thereafter, and the population declined to 59, but it was soon on the increase again, aided by the last two major contributors to the population—two Italians who settled on the island in 1892. Two more immigrants came early in this century (this time from Ireland), and a couple of genetic contributions were made by transient sailors. The genotypes of the offspring of these individuals have been observed, and these late genetic contributions have been separated from the main core of the genealogy. Effectively, the island's population is descended from just eleven early founders, together with the two Italians, whose genotypes can be accurately inferred from those of their many surviving offspring.

By 1961 there were 268 islanders, all of whom were evacuated when the island's volcano erupted unexpectedly. Almost all were taken to the United Kingdom, where 243 were sampled for genetic, anthropometric, physical, physiological, and medical traits, in a comprehensive Medical Research Council study. The unsampled individuals were almost without exception young children under the age of three years, so what is available is information on a complete cross section of a population whose detailed and complex genealogy back to a few original founders is accurately known. If there is any population in which the current distribution of genetic traits will provide clear information about ancestral types, it has to be that of Tristan da Cunha. Unfortunately, the genetic systems that could be studied in 1961 were few compared to those that can be analyzed today. Individuals were typed for seven red-cell blood-group systems. Although a few enzyme systems were analyzed in a follow-up study in 1972, a complete

Figure 27. Marriage relationships among the early founders of Tristan da Cunha. Reprinted from Thomas and Thompson 1984 (with numbers, not names).

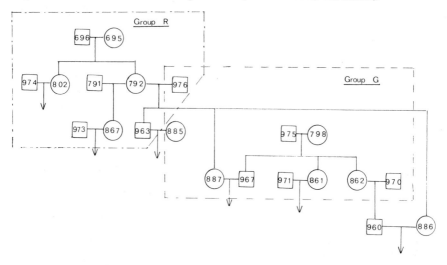

Table 26. Origin and number of descendants of the founders of Tristan da Cunha

Founder	Origin	Current number of descendants
Group R:		
974	England	144
696 ⎫ 695 ⎭	St. Helena	242
973	The Netherlands	177
791	St. Helena	177
Group G and R:		
976	England	235
Group G:		
970	U.S.A.	131
975 ⎫ 798 ⎭	Scotland ⎫ S. Africa (Dutch) ⎭	233
971	U.S.A.	96
885	St. Helena	171
Recent founders:		
994	Italy	71
995	Italy	48
795	England	14
866 ⎫ 793 ⎭	Ireland	89
796	—	2
790	—	1

Note: The definition of the founder groups is given in section 5.2.

population cross section was not then obtainable. A few medical genetic traits also were included in the original study.

By 1966 the islanders had all returned to Tristan da Cunha; they remain a small, enclosed, and isolated population of considerable genetic interest. It may seem that the history of these few individuals has been both precarious and unique, and that the final study, while an opportunity not to be missed, is nevertheless unlikely to yield any general conclusions. But the history of bottlenecks in population size, and of the resulting few contributors to a current small population, is probably typical of the history of many of the small isolated groups in which much of human evolution has occurred. The only difference is that the evolution on Tristan da Cunha has occurred recently, and thus its details can be accurately known. It is of considerable interest to find out whether the current data provide information about the types of genes the eleven early founders possessed and whether it is possible to infer precisely what alleles each has contributed to the current population. If, regardless of the original genes, the same current distribution is expected, then clearly inferences are impossible. Conversely, if inferences are possible, then the types of the genes of founders eight generations ago have affected the trait distribution of today.

5.2. Aspects of the genealogical structure

In addition to the advantages of having few founders and plenty of current data, the Tristan da Cunhan genealogical structure is important for making inferences about types of ancestral genes. On Tristan da Cunha almost any pair of individuals are related to each other several times over, and are descended from the same small set of ancestors in many different ways. Table 26 shows that the St. Helenan couple are ancestors of 242 of the 243 people sampled in 1961; another individual is the ancestor of 235; the original couple, of 233; while several other founders have over 170 current descendants. (Unless otherwise specified, the "current" population will refer to the 243 individuals sampled in 1961.)

The total population, living and dead, consists of over 700 individuals, but fortunately it is not necessary to consider them all. Some have no sampled descendants. More important, the genetic information on many of the younger members of the population is irrelevant to inferences about ancestors. If the *genotypes* (not simply phenotypes) of both members of a couple are known, then clearly the types of the genes carried by their offspring convey no additional information about the types of genes ancestral to the couple. (This, of course, is the basis of the sequential computational method and model specification described in section 4.6). The only individuals required for ancestral inference on the basis of genotype data are the *senior sampled members*: those individuals sampled in 1961 not having

Figure 28. A marriage node graph of the major section of the ancestral genealogy of the Tristan da Cunhan population sampled in 1961. *L** and *L*** are specific sampled individuals (see text). Reprinted from Thompson 1978.

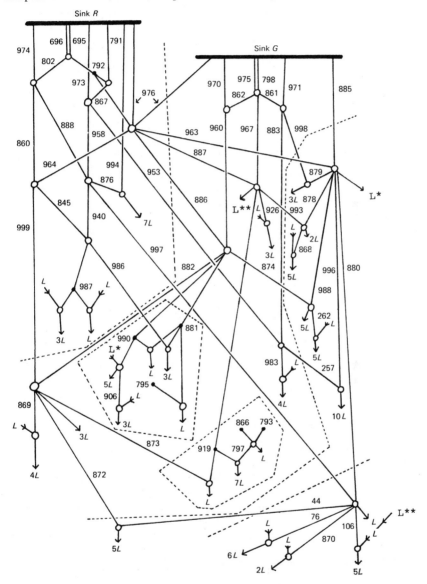

both parents also sampled. The genealogy then becomes relatively small and relatively simple; it is marriages between relatives still living in 1961 which reduce to chaos any attempt to draw the genealogy. Figure 28 shows the marriage node graph of this reduced genealogy, with $5L$ (for example) denoting a sibship of five individuals sampled in 1961. This genetic network, with genes entering through the founders and descending by repeated segregation to the present day, can also be thought of as an information network, with data entering through the points L and being driven upward to the founders.

Although the Tristan da Cunhan genealogy can be drawn, it is still large and complex. One family causes particular problems: individual 963 is a member of ten distinct interlocking loops connecting his six children to their spouses. These loops are then entangled with those involving other sibships. From the point of view of computational feasibility, it is fortunate that 963 is married to a founder. While many alternative lines of descent are necessary to provide information about ancestors, the complexity may make computations impossible. However, two pieces of good luck play a role here. Sampled in 1961 were individuals $L*$ and $L**$ of figure 28; one is one of the six children of 963, and the other also occupies a key place in the marriage node graph. These two women were aged eighty-three and eighty-five in 1961; but for their vigor and determination to be included, they might not have been sampled. Data on these two individuals make exact computations of probabilities feasible. Without them, either the operation would be very much more lengthy or some approximations would have to be made.

To obtain complete likelihoods for the types of genes of founders,

$$P(\text{data} \mid \text{genealogy, mode of inheritance,}$$
$$\text{hypothesized founder genotypes}) \tag{33}$$

must be computed for every possible combination of original founder types. This probability is then the likelihood for that combination; likelihoods of alternative combinations can be compared. However, with eleven founders of interest and three possible genotypes for each, there are 3^{11} such combinations to be considered. In working back through the genealogy to these eleven individuals, using the sequential method, it will be necessary to consider cutsets at least as large. In section 4.7, cutsets of eight or nine, and a combination of two successive cutsets jointly totaling no more than fourteen, were considered the computational limits. On the other hand, note that the sequential method provides the complete likelihood function with one computation on the genealogy. Functions L [equation (30)] are computed for all genotype combinations on a cutset of individuals. Working back through the genealogy, the final stage will lead us to the likelihood of equation (33) simultaneously for all genotype combinations in the founders.

Fortunately, the eleven founders fall naturally into two groups, each composed of six individuals. (In figure 27 and in tables 26–28 these groups are designated G and R in accordance with the notation of previous papers; the origin of this notation is not important.) One individual is in both groups which provides a very useful check on computations. The idea, then, is that, by entering prior genotype probabilities for the members of one group, it will be possible to work through the genealogy, accumulating information from current individuals upward to the other group, thereby obtaining a joint likelihood over all the $3^6 = 729$ founder combinations of that second group. Conversely, entering prior probabilities for this group may make it possible to obtain a joint likelihood over the founders of the first group. The question of what prior probabilities to assign is deferred to the next section. The two groups are marked in figure 27 and table 26, and figure 28 shows each set connected together to a single node at the head of the genealogy, which may be considered the final objective node of a cutset sequence. Thus, the process may be viewed as a sequential computation over the whole genealogy (section 4.6), the penultimate cutset being that of the connected six founders and providing the likelihood [equation (33)].

The procedure proposed above is computationally difficult, but it is feasible. One can work back to either of the two groups of founders without at any stage having to consider cutsets of more than eight individuals. That is, the maximum number of terms in any intermediate Q function or L function is $3^8 = 6,561$. In working from one cutset to the next, no more than a total of thirteen individuals are involved at any stage; $3^{13} = 1,594,323$. Since many of these 1.6 million combinations are in fact impossible, an efficient approach allows a full computation to be made.

5.3. Ancestral likelihoods for polymorphic systems

The system that has been most extensively analyzed by the above methods is the MN blood-group system. The two alleles, M and N, are codominant, and hence genotypes are distinguishable. Furthermore, the alleles are approximately equifrequent on Tristan da Cunha, as they are in many other populations of the world. While lending greater variety and interest to the current population distribution of these alleles, this equifrequency does not make ancestral inference easier. In general, the ancestry of rare alleles can be inferred with greater accuracy (see sections 4.4, 5.4, and 7.4), and a priori the chances of clear inferences from these MN data seem remote. Suppose prior probabilities of (0.25, 0.5, 0.25) are entered for the (MM, MN, NN) genotypes of those founders *not* in the cutset for the final likelihood. (This supposition will be justified below.) It is then found that, in fact, quite a lot can be said about the MN types of ancestors. In particular, both the Italians must have been MN. Also, although for each group

of six founders there are nearly 700 possible combinations of *MN* genotypes, in each case the most likely is some 50 percent more likely than the
next, and some 1,000 times more likely than the least likely but still possible
one. The problem is that it is difficult to discern any pattern in a list of 700
terms.

Consider first, therefore, the *marginal likelihoods* for each founder
of group *G*. That is, "average out" not only the founders of the other
group but all the founders other than the one of interest, using the same
prior genotype probabilities given above. Clearly, variation in likelihood is
lost by this averaging, but some information remains. Table 27 shows these
marginal likelihoods for all founders. Since only relative values between
the three possible genotypes are meaningful, the figures have been normalized to an *MN* value of 100. That is, for example, 885 is 1.48 times as likely
to have been *MM* as *MN*, but only 0.17 times as likely to have been *NN* as
MN. This means that 885 is over eight times as likely to have contributed *M*
genes as *N*. The two Americans (970 and 971) are also substantially more
likely to have contributed *M* genes, while the original founder and his wife
(975 and 798) are more likely to have contributed *N*.

These marginal values provide some indication of possible inferences, and it is now possible to consider the joint likelihood more construc-
tively. For example, 970 is not just more likely to have given an *M* gene on
average, but in *none* of the set of 10 most likely combinations could he
have contributed an *N* allele: in all he has genotype *MM*. Similarly, 885
and 971 are almost always *MM* in the set of most likely terms, occasionally, *MN*, but never *NN*, the opposite being true for 975 and 798. Individual 976 is much more variable. Thus, the "average" conclusion is borne
out by the likelihoods of the joint combinations. Further, it is possible to
make detailed inferences—for example, to distinguish between the *N* genes
contributed by the original couple and the *M* genes of two of their sons-in-
law (figure 27).

Suppose now that different prior probabilities of genotypes were assigned; the above computations could then be repeated. In addition to ar-
riving at joint and marginal likelihoods, one could average out *all* the
founders with respect to these same prior genotype probabilities, and what
would be computed is

P (data | genealogy, mode of inheritance, genotype probabilities),

or a likelihood for parameters of hypothesized genotype probabilities
among founders. The most likely values of such parameters could then be
found, and would provide the most easily justifiable prior frequencies under which to then compute joint likelihoods for the founders. Figure 29
shows the marginal likelihoods for group *G* and the overall probability of
all the data observed on the genealogy under a variety of *MM*-genotype

Table 27. Marginal *MN*-likelihoods of the eleven early founders at assumed *M*-allele frequency 0.5, each expressed relative to an *MN*-likelihood of 100

Founder	MM		MN		NN
974	80	:	100	:	104
696, 695	85	:	100	:	107
973	94	:	100	:	98
791	99	:	100	:	100
976	103	:	100	:	113
970	132	:	100	:	68
975, 798	74	:	100	:	114
971	125	:	100	:	78
885	148	:	100	:	17

Figure 29. The overall probability of all *MN* data, and the marginal likelihoods for the founders of group *G*, over a range of *MM*-genotype prior probabilities. Reprinted from Thompson 1978.

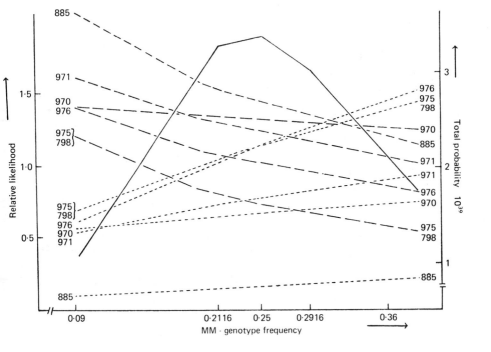

prior probabilities. If the *MM* probability is p^2, the corresponding probabilities assumed for *MN* and *NN* would be $2p(1-p)$ and $(1-p)^2$, respectively—that is, Hardy-Weinberg frequencies at *M*-allele frequency p [equation (1)]. The most likely p value is indeed found to be close to 0.5, giving the (0.25, 0.5, 0.25) probabilities used above. An alternative would be to use the frequency of the *M* allele in the current population, which is very similar (0.46). Of course, such an estimate does not take into account the genealogical relationships between individuals; the likelihood computation does precisely that. It is an oversimplification to assume equal and independent prior probabilities for the founder individuals. Independence is perhaps justified; the founders were not closely related. (Note that this is why the *parents* of the St. Helenan immigrants must be used rather than the individuals themselves.) Equality is more doubtful; the founders derive from very different source populations, in which *M*-allele frequencies vary appreciably. However, the precise origins of most of the founders are unknown, and allele frequencies that obtained 200 years ago are not available! The Hardy-Weinberg assumption is easy to implement, and seems an appropriate compromise.

Return now to the marginal likelihoods also shown in figure 29. Whatever the appropriate initial allele frequency, it must surely be in the range of 0.3–0.6. Whatever the frequency within this range, many of the previous conclusions hold. Individuals 885, 970, and 971 are always more likely to have contributed *M* genes than *N*, and over most of the range, 975 and 798 are more likely to have given *N*. Individual 976 is again clearly the doubtful case. Incidentally, note that *MM* likelihoods decrease and *NN* likelihoods increase as the *MM* frequency increases. This must be so. Genotype probabilities are entered for founders other than that (or those) on whom the final likelihood is derived. As the probability that those other founders carried *M* alleles increases, the likelihood that the founder of interest did so decreases.

The other group of founders, *R*, provides far less clear results. This can be seen from table 27, while the diagram corresponding to figure 29 consists of lines, mostly of rather low slope, all crossing in the center approximately at an *MM* frequency of 0.25. It seems that little can be inferred. However, on closer examination of the joint likelihoods, one finds that this group is as interesting as the other. These founders show a precise symmetry in their ancestry to the current population, in addition to the symmetries that always exist between the two members of a couple such as 696 and 695. The third most likely founder genotype combination is one in which 696, 695, and 791 all contribute only *M* genes, and the other three founders are *NN*. Exactly as likely is the combination in which the first three founders are *NN* and the second three are *MM*. This symmetry pervades the whole likelihood function. Wherever one possibility is that the six individuals have six specified genotypes, there is a precisely equivalent possibility of equal likelihood, which is obtained by switching the types of genes between the two sets of three. On averaging out to obtain marginal likelihoods for each individual separately, little variation remains. Thus, although it is not possible to make inferences about the individual genotypes in this group, a lot can be inferred about combinations. If certain individuals contributed M genes, it is almost certain others contributed N, and vice versa. This situation can also be viewed as a population bottleneck. These six individuals contribute to the current population mainly through just two couples (figure 27). While it is possible to make precise inferences about the alleles carried by each of the couples, it is obviously not possible to say which member of each couple carried which allele. The expanding ancestry of the two couples generates many equally likely alternative combinations.

5.4. The origins of rare alleles

At the other extreme from the MN blood types are the rare alleles present in the Tristan da Cunhan population. While it would be possible to trace the ancestry of these alleles using the biased recursive methods of section 4.4, it is here feasible to construct a substantial part of the complete ancestral likelihood, taking fully into account the individuals not carrying the allele of interest. Indeed, one of the attractions of the Tristan da Cunhan genealogy is that it enables one to make comparisons between alternative approximations and the full solution.

Some of the alleles that are infrequent on Tristan da Cunha are not rare in the world at large. For example, one rhesus allele, common in African populations, is here present in only one family, and can be traced to one of the Italian immigrants. Of greater interest, perhaps, is the B allele of the ABO blood-group system described in section 1.3. There are not many B-type genes on Tristan da Cunha; they show a frequency similar to that in European populations, and very much less than the 15–20 percent that is usual in African populations. One problem with a system such as ABO is that genotypes are not observable. An individual with blood type B may be of genotype BB or BO. However, partition of the ancestral and current populations by the senior sampled members enables one to analyze the data much as before. Using the data on current individuals, one can infer the ABO genotypes of these senior individuals, absolutely in most cases, and as a likelihood over two alternatives in a few. These inferred types can then be used in the derivation of ancestral likelihoods. Thus, whether genotype or phenotype data are available, the partition between current and ancestral genealogy remains a useful procedure.

The study of the B-allele distribution and ancestry raises interesting questions about the structure of ancestral likelihoods, the possibilities for and accuracy of approximations in computation, and the effects of dominance patterns and of a multiplicity of alleles upon inferences (Thomas 1984). However, in practical terms the results are clear and can be stated briefly. It is likely that one B-type gene entered with a recent immigrant, and that the only other was contributed by 885, the immigrant of 1863. Although the B-allele frequency is now typical of European populations, before 1863 it may have been entirely absent from the population. In a small population, chance events can have far-reaching effects.

Another rare trait on Tristan da Cunha is a recessive form of *retinitis pigmentosa*, an eye defect that eventually leads to blindness. This medical problem is perhaps of more immediate interest and practical importance than the ancestry of blood-type alleles. Four members of the 1961 population were affected, one of them being the grandparent of two others and the child of a brother-sister mating. There is no evidence of the trait's occurrence in earlier generations. Besides confirming the recessive character of this trait, these facts suggest that there may well have been only one copy of the allele—a_1, say—among the island's founding population. Given the rarity of the trait, it would in fact be surprising were there more. This one gene must therefore have descended by repeated segregations to each of the six distinct parents of the four affected individuals, and these six must all be heterozygous carriers (figure 30). There are presumably other carriers in the population. Thus, it is of practical interest to locate the origin of the a_1 allele, and hence determine the families most at risk in the current population.

It should be noted that if there was only one original copy of the allele, it must have been carried either by a member of couple (792, 976) or couple (975, 798), since only these four are ancestors of the necessarily carrier parents. Tracing the ancestry of only the four affected individuals suggests that 792, the immigrant daughter of couple (696, 695), may be the origin, but this conclusion is biased by the fact of her major genetic contribution to all current individuals. Ancestral likelihoods must be based as well on the normal phenotypes of the 238 individuals of the 1961 population of whom she is also an ancestor.

Since the trait is recessive, genotypes are not observable. This complicates the computation of likelihoods considerably. With regard to the data on affected individuals, there are three couples among the senior sampled members (figure 30) in each of which at least one member must have carried the a_1 allele. The problem can therefore be divided into eight cases, corresponding to each combination of three individuals who are assumed to be carriers of the allele. In each case no assumption is made about the other member of the couple: they may or may not be carriers with probabilities given by the relevant computation. (One, 990, is in fact necessarily a carrier, since he is a parent of an affected individual.) However, this is far from the complete solution. First, different trios of individuals among the

Figure 30. Obligatory carriers of the retinitis pigmentosa allele, and their parents. The genealogy shows only the cases and relevant interrelationships; normal individuals have been omitted. The three couples—*a* (213, 990), *b* (983, 52), and *c* (20, 19)—are discussed in the text. As usual, squares denote males and circles denote females; the same markings and labeling within symbols apply to both. A symbol with two markings (horizontal line plus inner circle) denotes an individual who has both the designated properties.

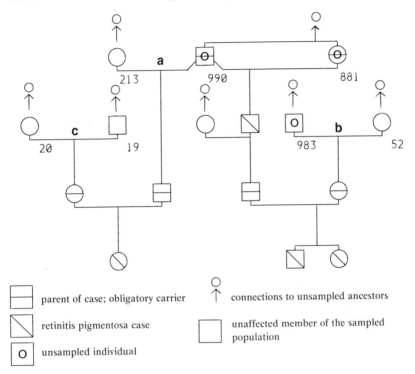

three couples have differing joint probabilities of being carriers, these probabilities depending also on the hypothesized origin of the allele. These must be taken into account in assessing the weight to be given to each of the eight cases. For example, 213 is *less likely* than 990 to have been the carrier giving rise to their grandchild case, since (apart from the fact that 990 is necessarily a carrier, being the parent of a case) a single gene carried by him could descend to all four cases. However, 213 is also *less probable* than 990 to have carried a_1 when the rarity of the a_1 allele and the joint ancestry of this and the other two couples is analyzed.

Likelihoods cannot be based upon the ancestry of affected cases alone; the normality of the remainder of the adult population also must be incorporated. Previously, the genotypes of the senior sampled members provided likelihoods on their parents. Thus, to compute overall likelihoods exactly as for the MN genotypes, likelihoods for the a_1a_1, a_1a_2, and a_2a_2 genotype combinations in the parents of senior sampled members are first required. These can be approximated by likelihoods computed on the basis of the normality of their descendants, disregarding the fact that these same individuals are also the descendants of other senior sampled members. Qualitatively, an ancestor with many normal descendants is less likely to have been an a_1a_2 carrier than one who has few, and on whom there is thus little information. For further discussion of this type of approximation see sections 7.3 and 7.4; its use in the Tristan da Cunhan analyses was an earlier one that I had not recollected until restudying the original computations. The effects of the approximation were compared with cruder assumptions in which only data on the senior sampled members were included, first as unaffected (not a_1a_1), and second as a_2a_2 noncarriers. The likelihoods differed of course, but relative likelihoods differed little, and qualitative conclusions were unaltered.

In order to compute marginal likelihoods for each founder, some assumptions regarding the a_1 allele frequency are required. In fact, some of the prior likelihoods for the parents of senior sampled members also require a probability for the types of genes of spouses (figure 31). Although rare in most populations, the allele was present in the set of eleven Tristan da Cunhan founders, and thus had a "frequency" of at least 1/22. Its crude frequency in the current population may be at least as large. The assignment of a prior probability among founders must be largely arbitrary. A small value is required in order that many origins not be hypothesized for the allele, and also in order that normality of almost all current descendants not be overweighted. (Recall that even including only those individuals old enough for reliable diagnosis, many will be counted several times over as the descendants of different couples among the parents of senior sampled members.) On the other hand, a negligible frequency will disallow the possibility of origin in other than those individuals ancestral to all obligatory carriers. In practice, several frequencies were experimented with, but the results presented here assume an allele frequency of 0.01.

Subject to all the above provisos and approximations, results are presented in table 28. While undue reliance should not be placed upon the quantitative value, there are several clear qualitative conclusions. It is on the order of 1,000 times more likely that the gene descends via 990 than via 213, and the most (a posteriori) probable carrier trio is (990, 983, 19), although this does vary with the hypothesized original ancestral carriers. Overall, the most likely origin is not a parent of 792 (that is, 695 or 696) but a member of the couple (975, 798). This couple is substantially more likely to have carried the allele than either the couple (695, 696) or the individual 976, but these remain possibilities. It is also of interest that 971 and 973 show nonnegligible although smaller likelihoods of having been carriers.

Figure 31. A schematic diagram of a section of the genealogy in figure 30 showing how current data are used to provide initial likelihoods for the parents of senior sampled members. Two such parental couples, *a* and *b*, are shown. As usual, squares denote males and circles denote females; the same markings and labeling within symbols apply to both.

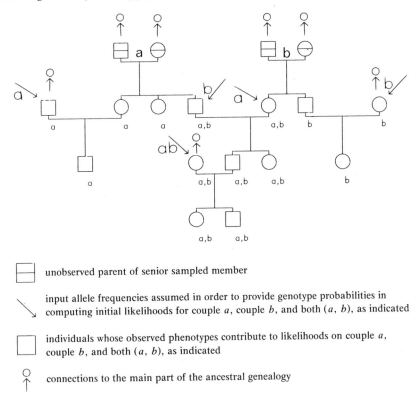

☐ unobserved parent of senior sampled member

input allele frequencies assumed in order to provide genotype probabilities in computing initial likelihoods for couple *a*, couple *b*, and both (*a*, *b*), as indicated

☐ individuals whose observed phenotypes contribute to likelihoods on couple *a*, couple *b*, and both (*a*, *b*), as indicated

connections to the main part of the ancestral genealogy

These two founders are grandparents of 983, but ancestors of neither 990 nor 213. Neither could be the sole origin. Individual 973 was the son-in-law of 792, and if he were a carrier, one of the couple (975, 798) would most likely have been a carrier also. Individual 971 was the son-in-law of (975, 798), and if he were a carrier, 792 and hence one of (695, 696) would most likely have been one as well. Thus, these subsidiary possibilities do not help resolve the main question, that of the origin of the allele.

Although the original obvious possibilities remain open, this analysis does enable some justifiable comparisons of alternative hypotheses of origin to be made. It is of particular interest that couple (975, 798) appears to be a more likely origin than couple (792, 976), which is ancestral to 242 of the current population. It is also relevant that the two alternatives provide somewhat different carrier probabilities for some members of the current

Table 28. Likelihoods for the origin of the retinitis pigmentosa allele

Assumed carrier in the parent couple (see fig. 30)			Relative likelihoods, including weighting by prior probability, of the carrier combination conditional upon each ancestral hypothesis				
a	*b*	*c*	696 695	976	975 798	971	973
990	52	20	1,335	593	943	368	350
990	52	19	670	1,644	2,674	482	128
213*	52	19	3	9	1	~0	~0
213	52	20	9	4	1	1	~0
213	983	20	5	1	~0	~0	1
213	983	19	3	1	1	1	1
990	983	20	2,429	347	950	316	1,103
990	983	19	1,142	491	3,296	555	420
Overall total			5,596	3,090	7,866	1,723	2,003
Overall ratio			71	39	100	22	25

*Since 990 is necessarily a carrier (fig. 30), those combinations in which 213 is so assumed have low likelihood. In most cases the prior probability also is low.

population. This means that future cases, if they arise, could give further information. It also means that beyond determining the crude values for normal offspring of obligatory carriers, for example, one should treat carrier probabilities with caution.

5.5. Gene extinction and survival

As described in section 4.8, ancestral likelihoods also provide probabilities of extinction of specified sets of ancestral genes. A long list of 3^6 ($= 729$) extinction probabilities for each group of six founders has little impact as it stands. There have therefore been several attempts to transform these probabilities to give a more meaningful picture of the genetic structure of the current population. One aspect is the dependence between the extinctions of genes in different founders or sets of founders. Given the ancestral genealogy, the survival of any given set of founder genes decreases the survival probability of other founder genes at the same locus. Conversely, extinction of certain genes decreases the extinction probabilities of others, or may even preclude their extinction. Some genes survive in the current population. A measure of such dependencies is the covariance between the events of extinction of different subsets of founder genes (see appendix 1). Such covariances may be readily computed within any set of founders for which a list of extinction probabilities of all subsets of the genes is available. Such covariances are small, since most extinction probabilities are so in any case and the dependence is a second-order effect [see appendix 1, equation (63)]. Relative to the possible bounds, however, survival of some founder genes has a large effect on the probability of survival of others. The patterns of dependence in extinction of the autosomal genes within group G and group R of the founders of Tristan da Cunha have been analyzed by Thompson (1979).

A more immediate and obvious question is how many distinct founder genes actually survive in the current population. For any given autosomal or X-linked locus, the probability distribution of numbers of surviving genes can be obtained from the joint extinction probabilities. The method is described by Thomas and Thompson (1984). These are probabilities based on the genealogy alone; in theory the current distribution of alleles also provides such information about the particular locus involved, but in practice the additional information is negligible for most loci. In some extreme cases of polymorphic systems, the variety (or lack thereof) in surviving allelic types may convey additional information on the number of distinct genes. On the other hand, for a system such as the MN blood types, the types and numbers of genes are confounded, and it is the types rather than the numbers that determine the current genotype distribution. To take an extreme example, suppose that everyone in the current population were of genotype MM. This would seem to indicate that for this locus rather few original genes survive, but the prime conclusion would simply be that the original genes were of type M.

To summarize only the results for the autosomal case, the probability that both genes of founder 976 survive is 0.81. If both survive, it is then most probable that seven of the ten genes in the five other founders of group G survive, compared to only five of the ten of group R. In this sense group G is more strongly represented than group R in the current population, although in terms of expected genetic contributions the difference is slight (44 percent to 41 percent if 976's contribution is divided equally between the two groups). Each group contains just one founder who contributes through only one child, and thus, necessarily, at least one gene of each group is lost. However, at least six genes of the twelve of group G (including 976) survive, whereas it is possible that only four of the twelve of group R (including 976) do so. In sum, at least nine of the twenty-two autosomal genes at any autosomal locus must be present in the sampled population; at most, thirteen are extinct. The largest probability is that fourteen are present and eight are extinct, but it is only slightly less probable that fifteen are present (see figure 32). The distribution is somewhat skewed toward smaller numbers of surviving genes, or toward larger numbers of *extinct* genes; note that figure 32 counts extinct genes. Many similar and

Figure 32. Probability distributions of the number of extinct genes at an autosomal locus: (*a*) extinct *G* genes; (*b*) extinct *R* genes; (*c*) extinct founder genes. Reprinted from Thomas and Thompson 1984.

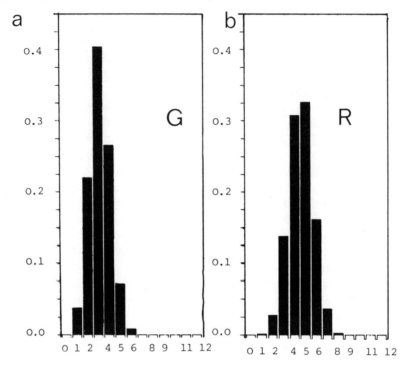

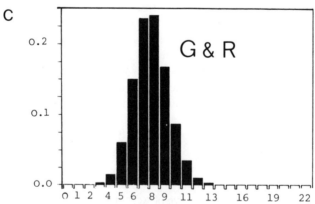

more detailed summaries of the pattern of surviving genes can be made; perhaps the major purpose of such a summary is to reemphasize the loss of genetic variability to be expected in a small and isolated population over a period of only 130 years.

5.6. Further reading

The original study of the Tristan da Cunhans was carried out under the auspices of the Medical Research Council, London. Lewis (1963) describes the scope of the study. Many of the early analyses of genetic and genealogical data were done by Professor D. F. Roberts and co-workers. Roberts (1971) gives many more details of the history than have been included in this chapter, and describes the demographic structure of the population as well as the basis for the reconstruction of an accurate and reliable genealogy. A detailed study of ancestral inference for the MN blood types and for the retinitis pigmentosa allele is given by Thompson (1978), the dependence between founders in the survival of their genes is analyzed by Thompson (1979), and Thomas and Thompson (1984) discuss the distributions of surviving autosomal and X-linked genes. Thomas (1984) gives a more detailed mathematical analysis of the form of ancestral likelihoods, using the B allele on Tristan da Cunha as an example.

6. Genetic Models for Pedigree Analysis

6.1. Models with discrete genotypes

The inference of the mode of inheritance of traits from genetic data is the remaining area of pedigree analysis to be considered. Section 4.5 provided a general specification of genetic models in terms of population distributions of genotypes, of transmission from parents to offspring, and of penetrance. The unknown parameters of this specification can, in principle, be estimated by computing

$$P(\text{observed data} \mid \text{hypothesized parameters, specified genealogy}), \quad (34)$$

where the data are the phenotypes for the trait whose mode of inheritance is to be estimated, these phenotypes being observed in the individuals of a set of genealogies whose structure is known. The computational problem is therefore the same as that of chapters 4 and 5. However, there are many problems in choosing a suitable class of models within which to make estimates in any practical situation, and it is necessary first to obtain some overview of the range of models available.

Although analyses of data are usually less clear-cut for quantitative traits than for qualitative ones, there need not be any essential differences in the underlying genetic model. Both can be modeled, for example, by a single Mendelian autosomal locus. The penetrances (probabilities of phenotype given genotype) are a discrete set of probabilities for qualitative traits, and are a function of a continuous variate for continuously varying quantitative traits, but this has no effect on the method of likelihood computation. There are, however, problems of the choice of the appropriate form of function in the continuous case. It may be convenient to specify, for each given discrete genotype, normal distributions of phenotype with given mean and variance (figure 33), but the normal form is not necessarily the true one. By transforming the data, one can achieve a mixture of normals from any form, and any form of distribution can be made to appear a mixture. There is a considerable degree of arbitrariness in the specification within which such estimates are made, and there are resulting ambiguities in the conclusions reached.

One classic model for a quantitative trait is the linear model for a single multiallelic locus. Consider alleles $a_1, \ldots, a_s$ with population frequencies $p_1, \ldots, p_s$ ($\Sigma_{i=1}^{s} p_i = 1$), in an infinite random-mating population (see section 1.4). The value of a quantitative trait in an individual of genotype $a_i a_j$ is assumed to be

$$X(a_i a_j) = M_{ij} + E,$$

Figure 33. A Mendelian autosomal locus controlling a quantitative trait through penetrance distributions defined for each discrete genotype

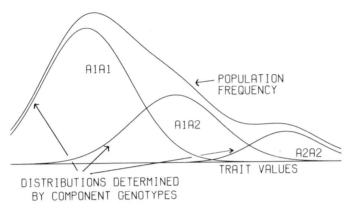

where E is a random environmental contribution of mean zero, constant variance over genotypes, and statistically independent of the genetic contribution M_{ij}. The genetic mean M_{ij} is then partitioned into

$$M_{ij} = m + c_i + c_j + d_{ij}, \tag{35}$$

where m = the overall mean of the M_{ij} weighted by population genotype frequencies

$$= 2 \sum \sum_{i < j} M_{ij} p_i p_j + \sum_{i=1}^{s} M_{ii} p_i^2 = \sum_i \sum_j p_i p_j M_{ij}$$

and c_i = the average increase in M_{ij} due to carrying allele a_i

$$= \sum_{j=1}^{s} p_j M_{ij} - m, \qquad (\sum_{i=1}^{s} p_i c_i = 0).$$

There are no implicit assumptions in the linear model [equation (35)], for the set of values $d_{ij} = M_{ij} - m - c_i - c_j$ allow an arbitrary form of M_{ij}. Note that $\sum_{i=1}^{s} p_i d_{ij} = \sum_{j=1}^{s} p_j d_{ij} = 0$. The population variance of the trait is

$$\begin{aligned}
\text{var}(X) &= \sum_i \sum_j p_i p_j (m + c_i + c_j + d_{ij})^2 - m^2 + \text{var}(E) \\
&= 2 \sum_{i=1}^{s} p_i c_i^2 + \sum_i \sum_j p_i p_j d_{ij}^2 + \text{var}(E) \\
&= V_A + V_D + V_E,
\end{aligned}$$

defining these three parameters as the three terms of the equation on the previous line. Covariances between noninbred relatives also are expressible in terms of these parameter combinations; V_A is the *additive genetic variance* and V_D is the *dominance variance* (Falconer 1981). Thus, although the initial model involves many parameters, analysis is possible in terms of a few parameter combinations, which can be estimated from the distribution of traits among relatives. In principle, this reduction of parameters enables one to make quite accurate estimates, although there are practical problems. Environmental effects shared by relatives inflate the covariances, and mating that is nonrandom with respect either to genealogical relationship or to phenotype also alters the usual formulas.

The next level of model complexity still retains discrete genotypes (figure 34). These are the multilocus models, where traits are determined by genotypes at several linked or unlinked loci (see section 1.6). Again, the traits may be either quantitative or qualitative, but the quantitative case involves too many parameters for precise estimates to be made. Models with linked loci more normally consider joint inheritance of qualitative traits, or perhaps an association in segregation between a quantitative trait

Figure 34. A schematic diagram of the range of genetic models available for use in pedigree analysis

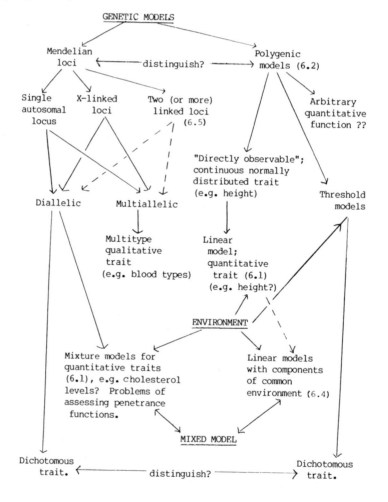

and qualitative markers. Models with linked loci will be most useful where the inheritance of some traits is determined by simple, precisely known, single-locus models and it is hypothesized that another trait is determined by loci linked to these. Any unknown linkage parameter in the transition probabilities from parents to offspring makes information on any unknown penetrance probabilities far less precise.

6.2. Polygenic models

A second range of models is provided by "genotypes" that are not discrete but take values in a continuum. Some forms of this model can be derived as limiting forms of models with large numbers of loci, each with a small effect on the trait of interest; hence the name *polygenic model*. However, its parameters and properties are sufficiently different from the case of discrete loci undergoing Mendelian segregation that it is simpler to specify it as a distinct model without reference to the hypothetical component loci. Each individual has a polygenic value, or polygenotype, P, which in the population is normally distributed with a certain population variance, v_P. The polygenic value for a child, given those of his parents, also is normal, with the mean being a linear combination of the parental values, and with variance v_T, say (the transition variance). The simplest model is that individual B with parents M and F has

$$P_B = (1/2)(P_M + P_F) + e_B.$$

Here e_B is normal, with mean 0 and variance v_T. If population variance remains constant [$\text{var}(P_B) = \text{var}(P_M) = \text{var}(P_F) = v_P$], and if spouses are independent with respect to the trait of interest [$\text{cov}(P_M, P_F) = 0$], this gives

$$v_P = (1/2)^2 v_P + (1/2)^2 v_P + v_T,$$

and hence

$$v_T = (1/2)v_P. \tag{36}$$

Further, sibs B_1 and B_2 have the same parents (M and F) but independent values of the transition variable e; their polygenic values P_1 and P_2 thus satisfy

$$\text{cov}(P_1, P_2) = \text{var}[(1/2)(P_M + P_F)] = (1/2)v_P.$$

Thus, as in the single-locus multiallele linear model of the previous section, certain variance functions of parameters arise in any analysis of data on related individuals. These few parameter values mean that the model can be a very powerful one when used appropriately. Note that equation (36) is an equilibrium relationship: in any finite population v_P must decrease with increasing inbreeding, and in the course of this process the relationship will be only approximate (Falconer 1981).

However, P itself is not observed; some specification of the relationship between polygenotype and observed phenotype also is required. For some traits (perhaps height is an example), one can effectively observe P, but in general a quantitative phenotype is some arbitrary function of P, with unknown parameters. Such a complex model is unlikely to be useful for inference. Qualitative traits can also be determined by a polygenotype. For example, all individuals with a P-value greater than a certain threshold may be affected with some trait, or probabilities of being affected may be an increasing function of P. As with the penetrances for discrete genotypes, these probabilities may depend on age, sex, or individual environment.

Within this class of models are the additive linear models, in which observed phenotypes are assumed to be an additive combination of polygenic value and independent environmental effects:

$$X = P + E.$$

Except where genetic and environmental effects are normally distributed in the population, this model causes inconsistencies in any attempt to apply equilibrium analyses of parameter values (see section 6.3 below). However, where phenotype is approximately normally distributed, and underlying effects also can be reasonably so assumed, the model is particularly tractable, for all joint distributions of phenotype or genotype among relatives take a multivariate normal form. The distribution is then specifiable by its mean and variance, and many methods of standard statistical analysis apply.

These models have the advantage that they can readily incorporate environmental effects common to several members of a family, and also assortative mating, where phenotypes of a married couple are not independent of each other:

$$X = P + C + E,$$

where C denotes common environmental effects. The difference between C-type effects and polygenic components is that only the latter are transmitted from parents to offspring. Clearly, an environmental effect could be not only common to several family members but also "transmitted" according to some distribution for children's values conditional upon values for their parents. Such an effect of cultural inheritance would operate effectively as a genetic component in terms of likelihood analysis of the model. These extra effects increase the amount of computation required, but not its complexity.

The *mixed model* includes both discrete genotypes and polygenotypes in the inheritance pattern of the trait of interest. The usual generalization of the polygenic case is simply to add an effect for the discrete geno-type of an individual into the equation for phenotype determination:

$$X = Y_{ij} + P + C + E,$$

where Y_{ij} is some random or deterministic effect of genotype $a_i a_j$. The aim in considering this model is usually to attempt to distinguish from "genetic background" P "major genes" determining the inheritance of a trait. The standard statistical approach is to consider a model incorporating both ef-fects, and to test whether either of the two alternative genetic components can be dropped. This assessment is made on the basis of the difference in log-likelihood (see appendix 3) between the more general model and the more restrictive model. If the difference is slight, the simpler model can be deemed an adequate explanation of the data. However, the increased com-plexity of computational procedures, of the structure of the likelihood sur-face for parameters, and of the parameter space involved render the mixed model infeasible in most practical situations. An alternative approach to the detection of major genes is through linkage analysis; this is the ap-proach taken in section 6.5.

6.3. Population constraints on parameters

In fitting a model to data, parameters of transmission, population, and penetrance may in principle be fitted without constraint on their joint values. However, a fitted model that is not internally consistent is an un-convincing explanation of observed data, and explicit or implicit relation-ships between parameter values can also substantially reduce the dimen-sionality of the parameter space. For example, populations seldom exhibit genotype frequencies in exact Hardy-Weinberg equilibrium, but unless there are specific reasons for an alternative assumption it is sensible to as-sume such frequencies for the founder members of the genealogy. It is likely to be an accurate approximation, and reduces the dimensionality of this part of the parameter space from one less than the number of geno-types to one less than the number of alleles (since in both cases the frequen-cies sum to 1). More generally, populations are continually evolving, and are perhaps seldom in exact genetic equilibrium, but changes in the means or variances of genetic effects on a trait are slow, and it is plausible to take them as constant within a genealogy, unless perhaps the trait is subject to very strong selection.

Such equilibrium assumptions give rise to relationships between the different classes of parameters. A simple example was encountered above, where independence between spouses and constancy of variance implies $v_T = (1/2)v_P$ [see equation (36)]. The theoretical population genetics of complex models is outside the scope of this text, and the problem is men-tioned only to engender caution in applying complex models without first discovering their properties. A further indication of the type of interrelationship arising between parameters is obtained by considering the effect of assortative mating for a quantitative trait. Note that nonrandom mating with respect to phenotype can itself impose selection on a trait, due to restricted availability of mates, whereas nonrandom mating with respect to genealogical relationship changes genotype frequencies but not the expected frequencies of underlying alleles (see sections 1.4 and 1.6).

Assortment is determined by phenotypes, often in the form of a positive correlation—b, say—in the phenotypes of spouses. But phenotypes are partly determined by genotype, and the correlation in phenotype induces an a posteriori correlation in the underlying genotypes of spouses. It is the joint genotype frequencies of spouses that are the *population* parameters entering likelihood computations, but correlation in genotype is related to that in phenotype via the *penetrance* parameters of the trait. In the simplest polygenic model of the previous section, this "penetrance" effect is determined by the relative proportions of genetic and environmental contributions to the variance of the trait. The induced correlation between the polygenotypes P_M and P_F of spouses M and F is

$$bv_P / V \quad \text{(which will be denoted } b^*\text{)},$$

where v_P is (as before) the variance of the genetic contribution and V is the total individual phenotypic variance. Also, from the equation of transition giving rise to equation (36), a more general equation relating the parameters is now obtained:

$$v_P = \text{var}(P_B) = \text{var}((1/2)(P_M + P_F)) + v_T$$
$$= (1/4)(2v_P + 2b^*v_P) + v_T$$

or

$$v_T = (1/2)(1 - b^*)v_P. \tag{37}$$

Thus, *transition* parameters are also related to those of population and penetrance via this equilibrium assumption.

6.4. Computation of likelihoods

For discrete genotypes, the methods of section 4.6 provide a procedure for computation of likelihoods for specified parameter values. Determination of the values maximizing the likelihood, and more general investigation of the form of the likelihood surface, are more complex problems. One method that can be useful is the computation of first and second derivatives of the likelihood with respect to certain parameters. Consider the form of the sequential equations of section 4.5; the new accumulated conditional or joint probability on a section of the genealogy is a sum of products of previous probabilities; population frequencies, segregation functions, and penetrance contributions. For example, in proceeding from child A to parent B, incorporating data on a peripheral founder parent C (figure 35),

$$L_B(i) = \Sigma_j\{ R(j)\ S_C(j)\ \Sigma_k\ [T(k\mid i, j)\ L_A(k)\ S_A(k)]\}$$
[see equation (32) and example following].

Differentiating once with respect to any parameter gives an equation for the derivative of the accumulated probability in terms of the previously accumulated probability, its derivative, the other model-specific contributions, and their derivatives. For example, if θ were a segregation parameter in the above example,

$$\frac{\partial L_B}{\partial \theta} = \Sigma_j\left[\!\left[R(j)\ S_C(j)\ \Sigma_k\left\{\!\left[\frac{\partial L_A}{\partial \theta}\ T(k\mid i, j)\right.\right.\right.\right.$$
$$\left.\left.\left.\left. + L_A(k)\ \frac{\partial T}{\partial \theta}\right]\ S_A(k)\right\}\right]\!\right]. \quad (37)$$

Thus, first derivatives may be computed sequentially together with the total likelihood. In principle, the method may be extended to higher-order derivatives, but the sequential equations become complicated.

The incorporation of assortative mating into the likelihood computation is not difficult. The difficulty, as discussed in the previous section, lies in determining the model of assortment consistent with other parameter values, and the net effect of phenotypic assortment on the joint genotype distribution of spouses. This joint distribution can be expressed as the product of the separate probabilities, which arises with no assortment, weighted by some joint factor. In the sequential equations for likelihood computation, the genotypes of spouses usually appear together, and the only modification required is the inclusion of this weighting term.

The inclusion of several discrete and/or polygenic components, to-

Figure 35. A sequential computation of likelihoods and their derivatives

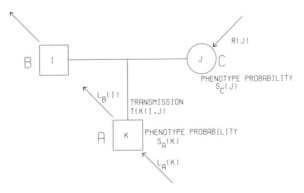

gether with possible effects of common environment, causes more fundamental problems, but the principle of sequential computation still applies. Previously, the accumulating contributions to the overall probability of observed data on a genealogy were probabilities given the discrete *genotype* of an individual or of a cutset of individuals. Phenotypes of individuals were dependent only via dependence in genotype, and given the genotype of any individual, data on those related to him via his parents were independent of data on individuals connected to him via his offspring. Now, several "attributes" can contribute to phenotype, and it is possible for them to be shared by several individuals and/or transmitted between them. These include contributions of common environment or of culturally inherited environmental components as well as the effects of discrete "major" genotypes and polygenotypes. Given the values of all these attributes, the genealogy can still be partitioned into independent sections (figure 36). Separate sequential equations apply to the transitions between different classes of attributes on different individuals. In principle, overall probabilities can be accumulated as before by considering at each stage cutsets, not now simply of individuals but (if necessary) of several attributes of each of several individuals.

This approach is seldom practicable on genealogies of any size or complexity. The limitations are due partly to the size and complexity of the cutsets that would have to be considered, since whenever information on the phenotype of an individual is to be incorporated, all relevant attributes must be jointly considered. In addition, where assortative mating is to be included, the phenotypes, and hence all relevant attributes, of (at least) the pair of spouse individuals must be considered jointly. However, the simple magnitude of the problem is not the main difficulty. A more serious problem is that many of the attributes may be continuous variates. There is no longer a finite set of possible values on which to compute the conditional probabilities of data on a section of genealogy, and the summations in the sequential equations become integrals. The two alternatives, neither generally satisfactory, are either to discretize the variates, using as many values as practicable, or to attempt to work with some parameterized functional form for the accumulated contributions to the overall likelihood.

There is one case where the latter is a feasible approach. If all attributes are continuous, with normal distributions in the population, and all transition, penetrance, and assortment functions are similarly of normal form, the joint distribution of any collection of attributes of any set of individuals and of probabilities of observed data on any genealogy section will be of multivariate normal form, determined by its mean and variance. Progressing through cutsets of genealogy, computing sequentially these means and variances, we return to the problem of the previous discrete, although still possibly very large, set of values to be considered. Note that

Figure 36. An example of a complex model: The mixed model with assortative mating and common sib environment. Reprinted, by permission, from *Current Developments in Anthropological Genetics*, ed. J. H. Mielke and M. H. Crawford (London: Plenum Press) (Cannings et al. 1980).

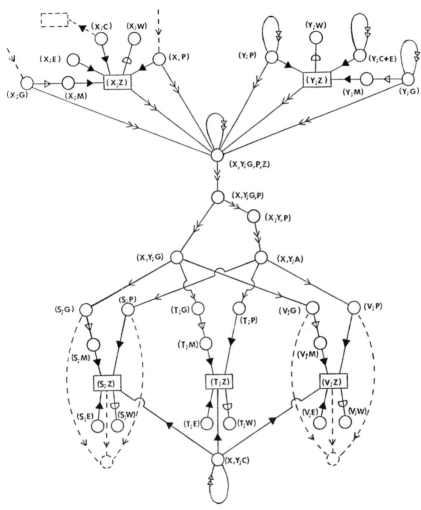

this method is not applicable to the mixed model; the contributions of genotypes undergoing Mendelian segregation destroy the overall multivariate normality. The net likelihood is a mixture of multivariate normal components, but the number of components is the number of possible Mendelian genotype combinations on the genealogy. Various attempts to simplify or approximate this mixture have been made.

6.5. Detection of major genes; linkage analysis

The location of genes on chromosomes and the genetic linkage arising in consequence have been described in section 1.6. Clearly, any single
locus whose alleles determine or have a major influence on the phenotype
for a trait must be located at some position on some chromosome, and thus
be linked to loci in nearby positions. By distributing a large number of
"marker loci" over the genome, one could locate single-locus traits. More
important, linkage to a marker locus would also provide clear evidence for
the single-locus nature of the trait of interest. In a genealogy, cosegregation of a trait phenotype of interest with alleles at a known marker locus
can only be the result of some causal effect of a locus closely linked to the
marker (or of the marker locus itself).

In principle, any known locus can be used as a marker, but few are
useful. First, the marker must be polymorphic, preferably with several alleles with nonneglible frequencies, for only parent individuals heterozygous at both loci provide linkage information (section 1.6). Occasionally, a
normally noninformative locus can provide a lot of information in a particular genealogy, due to an unexpected distribution of rarer alleles. Second, the pattern of phenotypic expression at the marker locus should be
straightforward. If inferences are to be made about a trait of interest, a
trait whose inheritance pattern will not normally be exactly known, it is
important that genotypes at the marker locus at least be clearly determined. If choice of marker loci is possible, an even spread through the
genome increases the chance of detecting some linkage for the trait of interest. On the other hand, if several markers are available and are themselves
closely linked, there is much greater power in the joint system to determine
the exact location of the trait locus relative to these markers. A new possibility in choice of markers is arising with the extensive work on DNA sequences and on polymorphic systems determined by restriction-fragment
lengths (Botstein et al. 1980), but as yet, red-blood-cell and electrophoretic
enzyme types remain the most frequently used markers. There are many
polymorphic systems whose locations on a wide variety of chromosomes
are known. Readers unfamiliar with the extent of this knowledge may find
it interesting to examine the review of Keats et al. (1979).

It is not possible to demand a specific mode of inheritance for the
trait of interest, nor even one that is precisely known. In fitting a genetic
model, it may be necessary to estimate jointly penetrance parameters or
allele frequencies with the recombination fraction. Where large genealogies are available this should not preclude the possibility of inferring linkage, but any uncertainty of genotype at the hypothesized trait locus will
reduce the information available for linkage estimates. Where possible,
preliminary estimates of other parameters should be made to prevent any
confounding of these estimates with recombination fractions from produc-

ing spurious, apparent linkages. For quantitative traits the problems are greater, for then trait-locus phenotypes are even more uncertain. Although tests of linkage of a quantitative trait with marker loci can still in principle be made, and such linkage would serve as evidence of a major effect from a single locus, in practice the power to detect such effects is small, and very large amounts of data would be required. Where a trait is genetically homogeneous, log-likelihood differences can be summed to combine information from several genealogies (see appendix 3). However, genetic homogeneity cannot be guaranteed. In different populations, different major loci could determine phenotypically similar traits, and where possible it is preferable to establish linkage within a single genealogy. For this, extended genealogies are required, but not necessarily complex ones.

Linkage involves the cosegregation of alleles at different loci, but the configuration of alleles on parental chromosomes may be unknown. In figure 37, for example, alleles a_1 and a_1^*, or alleles a_1 and a_2^*, may be on the same chromosome. This pairing is known as the *phase* of the configuration. Given certain parental genotypes, it is possible to divide the offspring into two sets, one of which is the result of recombinations and the other not, but it is not possible to establish which is which without knowledge of the parental phase. Thus, in nuclear-family data, the likelihood of a given recombination fraction r must always be the same as that of $(1 - r)$. Historically, therefore, studies have restricted attention to r values between 0 and 0.5, which have clear genetic interpretation. However, in an extended genealogy, substantial phase information may be available from knowledge of grandparental genotype and/or relationships between nuclear families. This information can increase the power to detect linkages.

This knowledge of phase is distinct from any possible observed association between certain marker alleles and trait phenotypes in the population at large. Linkage is neither a necessary nor a sufficient condition for such population association. In a small population such association may appear by chance, even in the absence of any causal effect such as selection, but the expectation is for no such effect, and associations are unlikely to be large. If there is linkage, particularly if this linkage is close, any association arising will decay only slowly, by a factor $(1 - r)$ per generation (section 1.6). Thus, in a single genealogy, a particular rare trait-phenotype is likely to be associated with a particular allele at any closely linked marker locus, for the ancestral copy of the allele determining the trait will be on the same chromosome as a certain marker allele and will tend to remain in conjunction (phase) with it. In a single genealogy, disequilibrium can be a useful indication of linkage but does not itself affect the likelihoods for cosegregation determined by the recombination fraction r.

Likelihoods for linkage are of the same general form as for any other model. The probability of the observed data on the genealogy is computed under alternative values of r, and values are compared by considering the

Figure 37. Examples of linkage analysis in which one parent is doubly heterozygous (the other, doubly homozygous for ease of identifying offspring chromosomes): (*a*) alleles a_1 and a_1^* are in phase; (*b*) alleles a_1 and a_2^* are in phase.

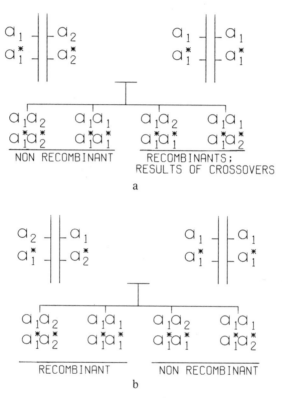

difference in log-likelihoods. The underlying genotypes are of course the joint genotypes at the two loci in question, and *r* is a parameter of the transition probabilities from parents to offspring. In fact, linkage analysis is one of the earliest forms of model-fitting by likelihoods, and so has evolved its own particular terminology and methods. The log-likelihood difference between any *r* value and the null hypothesis $r = 0.5$ of no linkage is referred to as the "LOD score" for *r*, and the value for that *r* maximizing the likelihood is known as the "LOD score for linkage." Unlike likelihood theory and analyses in most other contexts, LOD scores are almost always given using logarithms to base 10. These conventions are used in the example of the following section. (In fact, likelihood values obtained from a computer are likely to be given with a decimal exponent, and thus 10 is a convenient base for log-likelihood differences in most pedigree analysis contexts.)

6.6. Analysis of data in a Habbanite isolate

An example of the detection of possible major genes by linkage analysis is provided by the following analysis of dermatoglyphic data on a large genealogy of members of the genetically isolated Habbanite population. Previous analysis by Slatis, Katznelson, and Bonné-Tamir (1976) had suggested that single major-gene effects determined various common digital patterns in this isolate. Two large genealogies demonstrated the inheritance of an arch pattern on some digits. The larger of these two genealogies (figure 38) was considered by Anderson et al. (1979).

On this small set of individuals in a single genealogy, any attempt to fit a complex mixed model would be meaningless. There is no power to distinguish more than a few parameters. A simple single-gene model was

Figure 38. A pedigree analyzed for the mode of inheritance of a dermatoglyphic trait. Solid symbols indicate the phenotype "any arch." Reprinted, by permission, from Anderson et al. 1979.

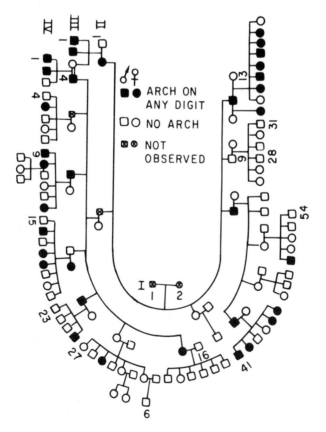

therefore first fitted. The phenotype "an arch pattern on any digit" was assumed to be determined by a single autosomal locus, with penetrance parameters, genotype frequencies, and segregation probabilities as given in table 29. The parameter p is thus the population frequency of the causative allele (a_1) for the trait, and Hardy-Weinberg equilibrium among founders is assumed. The parameter α is the penetrance of the trait in individuals either homozygous or heterozygous for the allele, and t is the probability that an individual heterozygous for a_1 passes on this allele to an offspring. The segregation parameter t was included to provide some check of the assumption of a Mendelian locus; the maximum likelihood over t was in fact obtained at $t = 1/2$, whatever the values of p and α.

Taking $t = 1/2$, two local maximums of the likelihood surface were found, the one of larger likelihood at $p = 0.05$, $\alpha = 0.95$, corresponding to a quite rare, nearly dominant, trait (figure 39). The other local maximum, at $p = 0.6$ and $\alpha = 0.05$, gives an unrealistically high allele frequency, and is of lower likelihood. Its existence does, however, indicate a general problem. High-allele-frequency, near-recessive traits are difficult to distinguish from rare, near-dominant ones. In the absence of independent knowledge of trait frequency, even a large genealogy may give little discriminating power, particularly where there is little inbreeding within the genealogy.

Although the model estimated is plausible, and the finding of Mendelian segregation proportions is encouraging, the fit of a single-locus model alone is unconvincing evidence for a single-locus trait. Only by computing linkage to a known marker can one obtain clear evidence. Linkage analyses for the trait with each of seven unlinked marker loci were therefore performed. Although blood-type data were available for only around 65 individuals of the 116-member genealogy, the interrelationships via the extended genealogical structure allow inferences to be made. Table 30 shows marker-allele frequencies previously obtained for this population by Bonné et al. (1970). Assuming these marker frequencies and the previously estimated values, $p = 0.05$ and $\alpha = 0.95$, likelihoods for the recombination fraction r were computed. Log-likelihood-ratio curves are shown in figure 40.

The maximizing values of r alone are not useful. It is necessary to consider the form of the complete function. It can also be illuminating to consider r values greater than 0.5. Such values provide a probabilistically valid model, even though they do not have a simple genetic interpretation. In an extended genealogy, the power of the data to reject values of r greater than 0.5 is a measure of the information about phase provided by ancestral relationships (see section 6.5). In figure 40, there are two loci (rhesus and P1), each strongly informative and providing information against linkage. The Duffy (F_y) and Gm systems also provide evidence against linkage, but are not so informative, as can be seen from the flatter curves and smaller

Table 29. The model for the Habbanite dermatoglyphic trait

Population frequency	Genotype of founder or offspring individual		
	p^2	$2p(1-p)$	$(1-p)^2$
Segregation probabilities for Unordered parent genotypes	a_1a_1	a_1a_2	a_2a_2
a_1a_1, a_1a_1	1	0	0
a_1a_1, a_1a_2	t	$(1-t)$	0
a_1a_1, a_2a_2	0	1	0
a_1a_2, a_1a_2	t^2	$2t(1-t)$	$(1-t)^2$
a_1a_2, a_2a_2	0	t	$(1-t)$
a_2a_2, a_2a_2	0	0	1
Penetrance:			
p (arch phenotype)	α	α	0
p (no-arch phenotype)	$(1-\alpha)$	$(1-\alpha)$	1

Figure 39. The bivariate log-likelihood surface for parameters p and α, showing the two local maximums

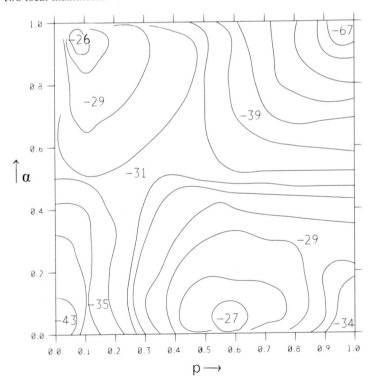

Table 30. Marker allele frequencies in the Habbanite population

Loci	Alleles present	Frequencies			
ABO	3	.15	.21	.64	
Rhesus	3	.48	.27	.25	
Duffy	3	.25	.17	.58	
Haptoglobin	2	.21	.79		
Gm	3	.23	.72	.05	
MNS	4	.33	.45	.01	.21
P1	2	.68	.32		

Source: Bonné et al. 1970.

log-likelihood differences. These four curves are also approximately symmetrical, which is to be expected in the absence of linkage.

The MNS and ABO results show statistically interesting features, but are unexpectedly uninformative on this genealogy. For the MNS system the maximizing r is 0.25, but this is not evidence of linkage, for (using logarithms to base 10) the log-likelihood difference between $r = 0.25$ and $r = 0.5$ is only 0.082. There is, however, some slight evidence against an implausible value of $r > 0.8$. In the case of the ABO system, the uninformative nature of these data leads not only to a very flat curve but also to two local maximums, one at $r = 0.78$ and the other at $r = 0.30$. The genealogical structure fails to provide phase information for this marker locus.

The locus of genetic interest is haptoglobin, for here the form of the curve, maximized at $r = 0.16$, shows evidence of linkage. The ratio of likelihoods at $r = 0.16$ and $r = 0.5$ is $10^{1.315} = 20.6$, and the ancestral data provide clear evidence on the phase in parent individuals, allowing r values greater than 0.5 to be rejected. To investigate this finding further, likelihoods were computed at different values of the penetrance parameter α. For $\alpha = 0.92$ the "LOD score" rises from 1.315 to 1.351, which was the maximum value found (figure 41). The point of major interest, however, is the insensitivity of LOD score and estimate of recombination fraction to changes in α, at least in the range $\alpha = 0.88$ to $\alpha = 0.95$. Although only relative values of the likelihood are relevant to distinguishing between alternative hypotheses, the absolute values of likelihoods also are of some interest. Where there are many data these are necessarily very small. Whereas for the dermatoglyphic phenotype alone, likelihoods are of the order 10^{-26}, those for the combined marker and digital phenotype are of the order 10^{-200}. This indicates a considerable number of informative segregations of alleles at the marker locus, as is indeed the case.

The question of the *truth* of an inference must always remain. This study is of particular interest in relation to others, in terms of both the

Figure 40. Log-likelihood-ratio curves for linkage analysis of arches: (*a*) ABO, Gm, and P1; (*b*) Rhesus, Duffy, MNS, and Hp. Reprinted, by permission, from Anderson et al. 1979.

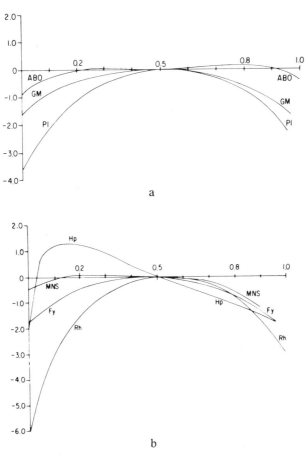

similarities and the differences of its findings. It confirms some previous indications, but other studies have suggested alternative hypotheses not here supported (see Anderson et al. 1979 for details). More recent studies on other populations also have suggested other inheritance patterns for dermatoglyphic traits, and other possible linkages. The particular study chosen for inclusion here is an informative one that contributed a substantial amount to the existing evidence. The results are as clear as can be expected for a study of this size, with likelihoods of expected magnitudes and likelihood surfaces of shape to support LOD score results and provide an overall consistent pattern of conclusions in which some confidence can be placed. It is through the combination of such studies that inferences be-

Figure 41. The variation of the maximizing recombination fraction, r, and of the LOD score for linkage between the haptoglobin and the dermatoglyphic loci, as the value of the penetrance parameter α is changed

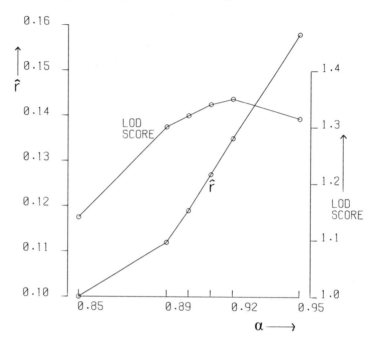

come accepted facts, but as yet the cumulative evidence is not conclusive, perhaps because the populations studied are genetically heterogeneous.

6.7. Further reading

Falconer (1981) provides a basic background on genetic models for quantitative traits. Updating his classic text (1960), he provides a useful introduction to this subject area, although it is directed toward animal breeding rather than toward the problems of human genetics. The more recent literature on genetic models is extensive; only a few papers will be cited here. The pedigree analysis approach is taken by Elston and Yelverton (1975), while the analysis of linear models has been considered in a series of papers by Morton and co-workers. The paper of Morton and MacLean (1974) is perhaps the most comprehensive of these, and provides other references. Cannings, Thompson, and Skolnick (1979, 1980) give details of computational approaches for likelihoods of complex models. Lange, Westlake, and Spence (1976) extend the analysis of quantitative traits on pedigrees, using multivariate normal distributions.

Linkage analysis has a rather separate, but no less extensive, literature. The classical approach is exemplified by Smith (1968), and Sturt (1978) describes a computer implementation of programs for the rapid analysis of linkage data. Ott (1977) has developed estimation procedures that can accommodate larger genealogies, while Smith (1975) discusses the problem of detecting linkage between a marker locus and a quantitative trait. Keats et al. (1979) give an up-to-that-date review of marker locus locations, and Botstein et al. (1980) introduce a new phase of development by discussing the use of restriction-enzyme variants for linkage studies in pedigree analysis.

The background to the population that provided the genealogy of section 6.6 is described by Bonné et al. (1970), and Slatis, Katznelson, and Bonné-Tamir (1976) describe analyses of dermatoglyphic traits in this population. Further details of the linkage study described in section 6.6 are given by Anderson et al. (1979).

7. A Study of Lymphoreticular Malignancies in Western Newfoundland

7.1. The study population

When extensive and complex genealogies come to attention, it is rarely the case that only a single question is asked. The problems of fitting genetic models, inferring ancestral origins of genes, and providing genetic counseling, are all likely to be involved, and their solutions interconnected. This chapter will investigate possible procedures for analysis, and illustrate both the scope and the limitations of pedigree analysis via a practical example. A new problem encountered will be that of inferences possibly biased by the fact that a data set is analyzed precisely because it displays certain phenotypic phenomena, these same phenotypic data being used as a basis for inference. Questions of ascertainment and sampling will be considered in more detail in the final chapter, but few studies can avoid this problem of bias entirely.

A study that combines many aspects of pedigree analysis is that of the occurrence of lymphoreticular malignancies in a group of three isolated Newfoundland communities. The West Coast Health Survey was undertaken by W. H. Marshall and colleagues at the Memorial University of Newfoundland after 21 cases of the diseases had been observed over a twenty-year period, 1954–1975.* A summary of the cases is given in table 31. Demographic and genealogical data were compiled, tracing the communities back to their settlement in 1820. Detailed genetic and medical data on most members of the population available in 1975 also were collected. The genealogical history of the settlements is an extreme case of a probably quite typical pattern. The initial founders were a couple, John-Charles and Mary (*J&M*), and their many children and grandchildren. Many later immigrants, both male and female, married into the communities, and the total genealogy has over 400 founders. However, the villages are extremely isolated and there has also been extensive intermarriage between the descendants of *J&M*, this couple remaining the major genetic contributors to the current population. In 1975 the three communities had a total population of 1,627 individuals, 1,521 of whom were descendants of *J&M*. The total genealogy comprises 4,028 individuals, 2,626 of whom are descendants of *J&M* (including the couple themselves). In the 1975

*This work arose out of visits to the Memorial University of Newfoundland in 1977 and 1981, and I am grateful to Dr. W. H. Marshall and others in the faculty of medicine for allowing me access to their data and for their continuing interest and encouragement. The data were collected with support from the Canadian Medical Research Council and the Canadian National Cancer Institute.

Table 31. Details of cases from the West Coast Health Survey, Workbook Number 2 (1977)

Case	Diagnosis	Sex	Year of birth	Year of diagnosis	Year of death
6765	Hodgkin's disease	F	1947	1954	1969
6731	Hodgkin's disease	M	1945	1965	1965
6790	Hodgkin's disease	M	1954	1966	1967
6086	Hodgkin's disease	M	1935	1966	1966
6800	Hodgkin's disease	M	1960	1968	1970
6019	Hodgkin's disease	M	1910	1970	1971
1005	Hodgkin's disease	M	1963	1973	1976
7262	Malignant thymoma	M	1958	1960	1960
6013	Benign thymoma	M	1901	1964	1969
6121	Lymphosarcoma	M	1925	1972	1972
6022	Lymphosarcoma	F	1908	1972	1973
7263	Lymphosarcoma	M	1962	1972	1972
1261	Chronic lymphatic leukemia	M	1907	1975	1975
7768	Acute lymphatic leukemia	F	1973	1976	1977
7638	Acute myelomonocytic leukemia	M	1890	1970	1970
6589	Rhabdomyosarcoma	M	1944	1964	1964
7238	Neuroblastoma	M	1962	1965	1965
1689	Retinoblastoma	F	1968	1970	1971
6500	Common variable immunodeficiency	M	1942	1973	1973
1141	Common variable immunodeficiency	F	1947	1974	—
1148	Common variable immunodeficiency	F	1952	1975	—

Source: Crumley 1977.

population the majority of individuals had received between one-eighth and three-eighths of their genes from the original couple (see table 32). The 1975 population is taken as the "current population" for the purposes of this study. Also included are those cases who were already deceased, but who would have been part of the 1975 population but for their lymphoreticular malignancies.

The broad questions are clear. Is this unexpectedly large cluster of cases attributable to environment, infection, or genetics—or to some combination of these? Is it significant that they originated when road builders reached the villages and provided the first prolonged contact with the out-

Table 32. Genetic contributions of the *J&M* couple to the 1975 study population

	Number of $1/16^{ths}$	Maternal contribution								
		0	< 1	1-2	2-3	3-4	4-6	6-8	8	Total
	0	106	1	13	64	50	97	27	20	378
	< 1	0	0	5	0	0	0	0	0	5
Paternal	1-2	31	3	18	59	7	37	0	0	155
contribution	2-3	98	0	28	84	33	90	29	4	366
	3-4	77	0	42	55	17	58	21	0	270
	4-6	84	0	23	88	31	73	23	28	350
	6-8	19	0	7	17	9	19	2	10	83
	8	1	0	0	0	0	12	0	7	20
	Total	416	4	136	367	147	386	102	69	1,627

Note: The numbers in the main body of the table are the numbers of individuals whose maternal and paternal contributions from *J&M* lie in the range specified. The numbers delimiting each range include the lower limit (except in the case of 0) but not the upper one; thus "1-2" means $1/16 \leq$ contribution $< 2/16$.

side world in 140 years? Did this contact bring relevant changes in diet and life style? Is it significant that all the cases originated genealogically from *J&M*? Are the cases even a homogeneous group? Are they manifestations of the same phenomenon, connected phenomena, or independent phenomena? Note here that the fact of 21 cases alone conveys little, for this is the reason for studying the population. The genetic, genealogical, and demographic distribution of cases must provide the information sought.

7.2. Preliminary analysis

Clearly, an immediate plunge into genetic modeling and pedigree computations is inappropriate. To obtain meaningful results, preliminary studies are required to determine a plausible framework of models for likelihood analysis. One method would be to examine the genetic and genealogical characteristics of control individuals matched with the cases for age, sex, and sibship size (Salmon et al. 1980), but this is not an ideal approach in this type of situation. First, to give meaningful results, the controls must be selected from the same population as the cases, which in this instance means from the same genealogy. Second, if controls are matched by sibship, then the sibships of cases must be avoided, and in the current situation this means severely restricting the choice of controls to the perhaps atypical peripheral parts of the genealogy and population. The major difficulty, however, lies in attempting statistical tests; cases and controls are interrelated, and the same ancestors and paths of descent that contribute to kinship between cases also contribute to relationship between controls.

A slightly different approach can, however, be useful. Taking the genealogical structure and current population as given, and also the fact of 21 cases as given, one can ask whether this set is "typical" of a random sample of the same size chosen without replacement from the population of 1975. A variety of characteristics of the set can be specified, such as age, sex, clustering within the genealogy, or descent from certain founders. In each case the probability that a random set of the same size would give a more extreme value of the relevant statistic can be determined. This is a version of Fisher's "exact permutation test" (Fisher 1956), and involves the usual problem of determining the relevant significance levels. However, means and variances can be readily computed in a potential sample of size 1,627, and with rather more computational effort, the third and fourth moments also. Together these allow one to make a reliable assessment of significance in a population of this size.

Table 33 summarizes the results of this exercise. There is no evidence of any age effect or sex effect in either the cases themselves or the pattern of their descent from the founders of the population. There is also no evidence that they are more descended from $J\&M$ than random members of the population, although the fact that the previously selected controls are significantly less so descended shows that there is some power in the genealogical structure to detect such an effect. However, this power is slight, due to the homogeneity of the current population in its degree of descent from $J\&M$. There is some evidence that cases, and particularly certain groups of cases, are clustered within the genealogy. There is also initially surprising evidence that some groups of cases are definitely less descended from certain early founders than randomly distributed groups should be; this result will be discussed below.

The first finding of constructive importance is the undoubted significance of bilateral descent from $J\&M$ (noted by Salmon et al. 1980). There is clearly some "recessive" type of effect, but this is not necessarily any indication of a single gene. That single-locus effects may be important is first indicated by the following observation. Among the cases are a significantly large number of individuals for whom the probability of descent from $J\&M$ of both the maternal gene (g_m) and the paternal gene (g_p) is greater than the product of the probabilities, these probabilities being computed on the basis of the genealogy for an arbitrary autosomal locus:

$$D_{JM} = P(g_m \text{ and } g_p \text{ both descend from } J\&M)$$
$$- P(g_m \text{ descends from } J\&M) \, P(g_p \text{ descends from } J\&M)$$
$$> 0 \text{ for a positive covariance in descent.} \tag{38}$$

Table 33. Exact tests of clustering and descent with respect to three founders and from a set, C_4, of the four children of *J&M* with the most descendants

Test criterion		Observed	Expected	Relevant 95% confidence limit
(a) Descent from				
	$J = 6501$	5.67	5.37	5.79
	6896	9.52*	8.76	9.48
	6996	7.62	7.42	8.14
	C_4	4.37	5.18	4.18
(b) Clustering in descent from				
	$J = 6501$	138	208	126
	6896	241	384	224
	6996	346	402	283
	C_4	360	384	333
(c) As in (b), but for HD/ID cases only				
	$J = 6501$	30	45	28
	6896	32	82	31
	6996	33*	86	47
	C_4	49*	82	63
(d) Descent from *J&M* unilateral		3*	8.1	3.9†
"low" bilateral‡		3 [1]	3.2	—
"high" bilateral		15* [9]	7.8	12.6
(e) Covariance in descent				
	$D_{JM} > 0 \ (N = 56)$	0	0.8	—
	$D_J > 0 \ (N = 264)$	7* [6]	3.6	6.4
	$D_K > 0 \ (N = 628)$	12 [8]	8.7	14.3

Note: Low values of the statistics indicate excess descent or clustering.

*A result outside the 95% confidence limit.

†Confidence limits between the observable integer values designate the appropriate proportions for randomization on the boundary for a test of exact size 95%.

‡Low descent includes individuals with up to ¼ of their genes expected from *J&M*, and high descent includes individuals with ⅜ or more. Numbers in square brackets denote the HD/ID cases.

That is, there is a covariance between the events of descent from *J&M* to the two genes of the individual (see appendix 1). For any ancestral set of genes, such a covariance in descent is a measure of the existence of intermediate bilateral ancestors of the individual, these ancestors being descended from the original ancestral gene set. If g_m is a copy of one of the relevant ancestral genes, then intermediate ancestors must also carry it, and the chance that g_p is also a copy is increased over the overall probability. In figure 42, for example, the ancestor B_2 receives from B_4 either a gene of J or a gene of M. If g_m descends from J, then the posterior probability that

Figure 42. A schematic diagram showing three levels of covariance in descent due to intermediate ancestors who are children, grandchildren, or great-grandchildren of J, giving covariance with respect to a single gene of J, both genes of J, and genes of the $J\&M$ couple, respectively.

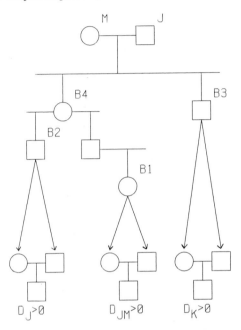

B_2 received a gene of J and not one of M is increased. (Indeed, if there are no other paths of descent, B_2 must necessarily carry a gene of J if g_m is to be such a gene.) Thus, the probability that g_p descends from J is increased over the overall probability that g_p descends from J, the single segregation from B_4 to B_2 contributing to both descents.

In this population there are three relevant levels of such covariance: in the descent from the genes from the $J\&M$ couple [D_{JM} of equation (38)], from the two genes of J (with analogous covariance D_J), and from a specified gene of J (say, K, with covariance D_K). Note that great-grandchildren of $J\&M$ may or may not receive a gene from $J\&M$, grandchildren must receive a gene of $J\&M$ but may or may not receive a gene of J, whereas children of $J\&M$ must receive a gene of J but may or may not receive the particular gene K (individuals B_1, B_2, and B_3, respectively, of figure 42). Thus, the three levels of covariance indicate, respectively, common ancestors among the great-grandchildren, grandchildren, and children of $J\&M$. The fact that individuals with positive such covariances are overrepresented in a group of cases—that is, exceed the expected number, given their level of bilateral descent—is evidence of single-locus effects descending "unbroken" on the paths to these intermediate ancestors. The total number in the population in the category with $D_{JM} > 0$ is small (table 33), but there are too many cases both of whose parents descend from the same grandchildren of $J\&M$ ($D_J > 0$), and perhaps also from the same child ($D_K > 0$). Further, it is here that a subdivision of the cases first clearly emerges, although it was already suspected from some of the earlier tests. Of the 7 cases with $D_J > 0$, 6 are cases of Hodgkin's disease (HD) or common variable immunodeficiency (ID); of the 12 with $D_K > 0$, 8 are cases of HD or ID; there are only 10 cases of HD/ID in all.

This question of the descent patterns from intermediate ancestors—in particular from the grandchildren of $J\&M$—can also be examined in reverse. Consider the set of ancestors of individual cases or groups of cases among these grandchildren. As shown in table 34, $J\&M$ had 71 grandchildren, G, 41 of whom have current descendants. Subdivisions of the current population are characterized by the subset of G from which they descend. Thus, for any set S of n current individuals, consider, for example, the mean number n_1 of members of G from which an individual in S is descended, and also the total number n_2 from which members of S jointly descend. Equivalently, but more conveniently, one can compute the "repeat frequency"—the mean number of times an ancestor in G is repeated as an ancestor of the group S. As before, the moments of the same quantities for a random set that is the same size as S, chosen without replacement from the current population, can be computed, and thus one can determine whether S is a typical random group.

As an example, consider first the set S_1, the 21 controls mentioned above. Individually, these controls descend from fewer members of G than a random individual should, a fact that again points to the difficulty of undertaking control studies in such a population. Given this low level of descent from G, and hence from $J\&M$, the controls are as a group well distributed among the members of G as measured by the repeat frequency shown in table 35. Consider second the set S_2, the 11 cases other than HD/ID. Individually, these are perhaps descended from slightly more members of G than random members of the population are, but not significantly so. Nor is their joint ancestry among the members of G atypical. There is no clear pattern, nor indeed evidence of any genealogical effect. This contrasts markedly with the set S_3, the 10 cases of HD/ID. Individually, the level of descent is not significantly high, but the repeat frequency is enormous. What contributes to HD/ID susceptibility is not descent from G in general but descent from a small specifiable subset of G, this being balanced by a *negative* effect of descent from other members of G.

This is precisely the expected pattern for a trait in which predisposition is determined by a single gene with recessive-type effects. It is also relevant here that all 10 cases of HD/ID are bilaterally descended from $J\&M$, for a single gene carried by one of $J\&M$ is, on average, carried by

Table 34. Descent from the grandchildren, G, of *J&M*: Number of grandchildren with d descendants

Grandchildren with	Children of *J&M* 7092	6597	6200	6606	7095	Three others	Total for all grandchildren
No offspring*	1	3	7	5	—	10	26
Offspring, but $d = 0$	1	—	—	—	—	3	4
$0 < d \leq 30$	2	1	2	2	—	3	10
$31 \leq d \leq 100$	3	—	—	4	2	1	10
$101 \leq d \leq 150$	—	2	—	2	1	1	6
$151 \leq d \leq 200$	2	4	—	1	1	1	9
$201 \leq d \leq 300$	1	—	—	—	—	1	2
$301 \leq d \leq 400$	1	1	—	—	—	—	2
$d = 584$	1	—	—	—	—	—	1
$d = 652$	—	—	1	—	—	—	1
Total number of sibs	12	11	10	14	4	20	71
Total number of current descendants	1,173	877	671	518	437	—	

*Only offspring residing in the communities are counted; thus, this line includes emigrating grandchildren, whose offspring reside elsewhere.

Table 35. Ancestry of chosen sets of individuals among the grandchildren, G, of *J&M*

Statistic	Results for set S_1 (controls)	S_2 (non-HD/ID cases)	S_3 (HD/ID cases)
Number (n) in group	21	11	10
Number (n_1) of ancestors in G per individual in the set:			
Observed	2.15	3.82	3.90
Expected (± 1 s.d.)	3.47 ± 0.40	3.47 ± 0.55	3.47 ± 0.58
Total number (n_2) of different ancestors in G	20	19	10
Repeat frequency (ν):			
Observed	2.25	2.21	3.90
Expected (± 1 s.d.)	2.78 ± 0.42	1.90 ± 0.39	1.84 ± 0.33

Notes: The definitions of the three sets are given in the text. "± 1 s.d." gives the one standard deviation limit on the expectation. The statistics shown are related by the formula $\nu = n \, n_1 / n_2$.

one-fourth of their grandchildren. Descendants from these grandchildren would be predisposed to the trait, while the other three-quarters would pass on to their descendants only "normal" genes. Further, recall that certain original founders, specifically spouses of the children of *J&M*, appear to give "protection" against the trait. This is now explained, were these noncarrier children of the original couple.

7.3. Likelihood analysis of Hodgkin's disease and immunodeficiency

Thus there is a priori justification for fitting a single-locus model to HD/ID, and fairly clear evidence that the other traits are altogether more complex and probably not closely associated. One can now proceed to likelihood analysis as in the previous chapters. The first conclusions are that, from the distribution of the affected individuals, if this is a single-locus trait, the allele was carried by John-Charles (or Mary) and by no one else who has made any substantial contribution to the current population; there was only one original copy. It also emerges that, statistically, HD/ID should be considered jointly as a single trait; this conclusion can be drawn from the genetic likelihoods, independently of any medical justification. The model to be fitted is of a single diallelic locus, and allele frequencies do not enter the problem, since a single original a_1 allele carried by John-Charles is assumed. There are, however, two penetrance parameters;

$$P(\text{affected} \mid a_1 a_1) = \alpha$$

$$P(\text{affected} \mid a_1 a_2) = \beta$$

$$P(\text{affected} \mid a_2 a_2) = 0. \tag{39}$$

In a more complex model, α and β could be age- and/or sex-dependent, but there is no evidence within the current data set that they should be. Nor would there be sufficient power to fit such a model meaningfully on this genealogy.

Computation of likelihoods over all α and β on the whole genealogy is not feasible, but it is so on the restricted core genealogy of the ancestors of the 10 HD/ID cases. This core genealogy is shown in conventional form in figure 43, and as a marriage node graph in figure 44. Even on the restricted genealogy, computation of the likelihood for each α and β combinations requires a separate lengthy computation. Evaluations are therefore made at only a limited number of (α, β) points, particularly those clustered around the vertex $\alpha = 1$, $\beta = 0$, since there is clearly a recessive-type pattern. In fact, maximum likelihood estimates are found to be $\alpha = 1$, $\beta = 0$, and the likelihood decreases quite sharply as β increases. The estimate $\alpha = 1$ may be an artifact of the section of genealogy considered: the ancestors of affected cases. The estimate $\beta = 0$ cannot be so, and initially, at least, is a surprising finding, which will be considered further below.

Figure 43. The core genealogy: The ancestors of affected cases, and their descent from the couple *J&M*. Reprinted from Thompson 1981*a*.

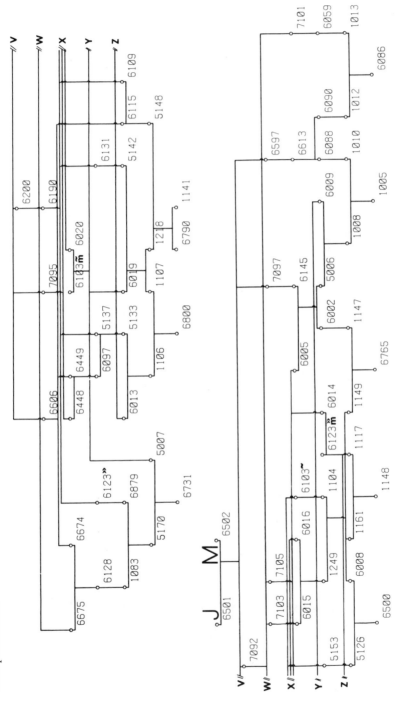

Figure 44. The core genealogy of figure 43 in marriage node graph form. Reprinted from Thompson 1981*a*. (Recent investigations have necessitated minor changes in this genealogy. Individual 7105 is the child of 7092, as shown, but by an earlier spouse. The [unnamed] fathers of 5126 and 1147 were probably the same man. The spouses of 6190 and 6200 were first cousins. These facts have now been incorporated into all computations; they do not alter previous conclusions.)

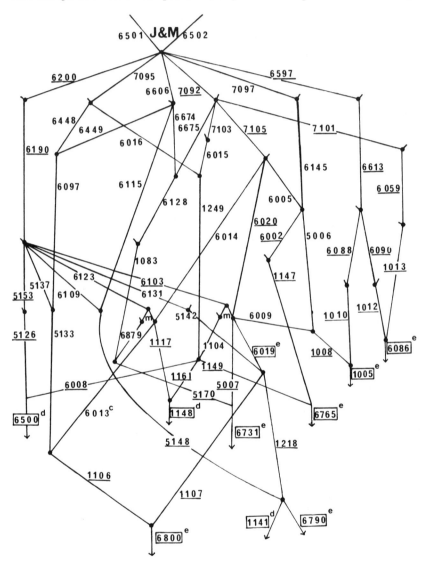

First, however, consider a child, B, of an individual in the core genealogy of figure 44, who is not himself in that genealogy as he is not an ancestor of an affected individual. He may have descendants who are (bilaterally) descended from $J\&M$, and who thus have differing probabilities of being affected if he is a_1a_1, a_1a_2, or a_2a_2. (In order to be conservative in our conclusions, in all computations non-case individuals who were not alive in 1975 were assumed to be of unknown phenotype rather than normal, even where their life histories indicate that they were probably not affected. Thus B may have been a_1a_1, even if $\alpha = 1$.) Observation of normal descendants in 1975 thus provides relative likelihoods that B was of each of the three genotypes. Of course, likelihoods for different individuals B are not independent, since they may be jointly ancestors of the same normal individuals, but as a good approximation these separate values can be incorporated into the overall likelihood. Again it emerges that if α is decreased from 1, or β is increased from 0, the likelihood decreases, and so the "simple recessive" conclusion derived on the core of the genealogy is confirmed by the periphery. However, the evidence $\alpha = 1$ is less strong in this instance than was indicated by the data on the core genealogy alone.

Why should the recessive finding ($\beta = 0$) have been unexpected? First, because of its simplicity. Normally the addition of extra parameters allows an increase in likelihood, even where the true hypothesis does not include them. That the maximum likelihood estimate is at the vertex of the (α, β) parameter space is convincing evidence for the simpler model. Second, because it clearly cannot be the correct model for all 21 cases, some of whom are only unilaterally descended from $J\&M$. It is only because the previous analysis justified a subdivision of the cases that this simple model will now explain the data. Third, there is the problem of the number of cases. For each member C of the study population, the probability that he carries two copies (q_C^{**}) and one copy (q_C^*) of a particular one of J's two genes can be readily computed. Then

$$P(C \text{ affected}) = \alpha \ q_C^{**} + \beta \ q_C^*, \tag{40}$$

and the total expected number of cases is

$$\alpha \ (\Sigma_C q_C^{**}) + \beta \ (\Sigma_C q_C^*),$$

where summation is over all members of the current population. For $\alpha = 1$ and $\beta = 0$ the result is 2.54, and were individuals independently descended from J, the observation of 10 cases would be incompatible with this. Thus, either $\beta > 0$ or the number of cases has been inflated by the dependence between individuals. That is, those children and grandchildren of $J\&M$ who chanced to carry the gene, also chanced to be the ones with large numbers of current descendants. This is clearly what has in fact occurred, and is, of course, an aspect of ascertainment. Had it not been these grandchildren who had many descendants, there would not have been 10 cases, and the population might not have come to attention.

This is reemphasized by the fact that if the gene is assumed to have been carried by each of the four grandchildren of *J&M*, who must, if this *is* a simple recessive trait originating only in *J*, have been carriers, then the expected number of cases is 7.8, and the observation of 10 is no longer extreme. For our single-locus model, the distribution of cases leads to the assumption of a single gene carried by John-Charles. This assumption is itself a form of "ascertainment correction," for only such genealogies will display many cases, but it is an insufficient one, for that event alone leads only to an expected 2.54 cases, even if $\alpha = 1$. It is thus of considerable interest that pedigree analysis detects the segregation pattern, and despite the fact of 10 cases gives $\beta = 0$.

7.4. Risk analysis and genetic counseling

The next stage of analysis, assuming now a single-locus trait $\beta = 0$ and $\alpha \leq 1$, is to trace the paths of the gene in the ancestral genealogy by computing the marginal probabilities that each ancestor is a_1a_1, a_1a_2, and a_2a_2, given a single initial a_1 allele carried by *J*, and the 10 homozygous a_1a_1 cases. These require several computations through the genealogy (see chapter 4) in order to obtain both "upward" and "downward" contributions to these risk probabilities for all individuals, but the answers shown in table 36 are surprisingly clear. Certain individuals, such as 6005 and 1104, show high probability of carrying the gene. This is not surprising; they are both offspring and parents of obligatory carriers. More important, other individuals, such as 1249, although ancestors of several cases, have high probabilities of the normal a_2a_2 genotype. Further, for given α, the extra contributions from the periphery of the genealogy via individuals *B* defined above also can be included. When they are included, previous results are confirmed; large risks increase and small ones decrease. In the extreme case $\alpha = 1$ the majority of paths are almost absolutely determined (see table 36), although for $\alpha < 1$ the pattern obviously cannot be quite so clear. So again the data on the periphery reinforce the findings on the core, and infer that the overall reconstruction is correct.

Of the offspring of *J&M*, there are three obligatory carriers, and two (7095 and 7097) who have nonnegligible probabilities of having been so, but were more likely not. This fits well with expectation, given that eight children of *J&M* have current descendants, seven having more than 250 each and thus providing substantial power to make inferences. Of the grandchildren, there are four obligatory carriers, and the analysis suggests only two more (7103 and perhaps 6675). Each of these six individuals has at least 80 descendants, and, in particular, three of the four with at least 300 descendants are implicated. Clearly there is both ascertainment bias and

Table 36. Posterior probabilities for the ancestral paths of the a_1 allele on the core genealogy in the case $\alpha = 1$

Individual	N_1	N_2	N_3	Core genealogy alone			Peripheral contributions included		
				a_1a_1	a_1a_2	a_2a_2	a_1a_1	a_1a_2	a_2a_2
7097	1	6	0	—	0.6	0.4	—	0.03	0.97
6145	2	4	146	—	0.4	0.6	—	0.01	0.99
6005	2	4	146	—	0.8	0.2	—	0.99	0.01
5006	1	5	14	0.08	0.47	0.45	0.05	0.30	0.65
6009	1	2	14	0.25	0.50	0.25	0.06	0.06	0.88
7095	2	2	181	—	0.591	0.409	—	0.06	0.94
6016	1	5	26	—	0.379	0.621	—	<0.005	~1
6448	1	4	39	—	0.306	0.694	—	<0.005	~1
6606	3	11	246	—	0.674	0.326	—	<0.005	~1
6449	1	4	39	—	0.316	0.684	—	<0.005	~1
6674	1	3	0	—	0.304	0.696	—	<0.005	~1
6115	1	8	36	—	0.406	0.594	—	<0.005	~1
7103	1	6	108	—	0.581	0.419	—	0.02	0.98
6015	1	5	26	—	0.373	0.627	—	<0.005	~1
1249	3	4	25	0.035	0.398	0.567	<0.005	<0.005	~1
1104	3	4	25	—	0.742	0.258	—	0.99	0.01
6109	1	8	36	—	0.796	0.204	—	0.99	0.01
6675	1	3	0	—	0.5	0.5	—	0.07	0.93
6128	1	2	25	0.038	0.288	0.674	<0.005	0.01	0.99
1083	1	2	10	—	0.202	0.798	—	<0.005	~1
6097	1	11	33	0.024	0.280	0.696	<0.005	<0.005	~1
5137	1	11	33	—	0.537	0.463	—	<0.005	~1
5133	1	3	18	0.041	0.395	0.564	<0.005	<0.005	~1
6123	3	10	196	—	0.923	0.077	—	~1	<0.005
6014	2	10	196	—	0.588	0.412	—	<0.005	~1
6879	1	2	10	—	0.967	0.033	—	~1	<0.005
6013	1	3	18	0.147	0.677	0.176	<0.005	0.01	0.99
5142	2	3	10	—	0.111	0.889	—	0.01	0.99
6131	1	4	47	—	0.385	0.615	—	0.03	0.97

Note: N_1 = number of offspring in core genealogy; N_2 = number of other offspring; N_3 = number of current descendants via offspring not in core genealogy.

information bias here. It is unlikely that there were only six carriers, even among the 41 grandchildren with current descendants, but those with few descendants may never be detected. On the other hand, the fact of ascertainment of this genealogy makes it likely that some grandchildren with exceptionally large numbers of descendants were among the carriers. Taking either factor (or both) into account, the conclusions are again so plausible as to give renewed confidence in the model.

One now arrives at the genetic counseling problem, which has both theoretical and practical aspects. The probabilities that both members of each pair of current individuals who constitute a potential parent couple are $a_1 a_2$ carriers can be computed. More generally, for $\alpha < 1$, the probabilities that they are nonaffected $a_1 a_1$ individuals also can be found. It is of interest that carrier probabilities are substantially altered by using the information on the complete inferred ancestral paths of the allele, both from those obtained on the basis of descent from J, and from those based only on the closest relatives. Thus, the analysis has certainly contributed information on the distribution of the gene in the current population, but this probabilistic information would hardly be helpful to the individuals concerned.

There are, however, four conclusions that may be of practical concern to the members of the population. First, there *is* a genetic immunodeficiency effect in this population, which has manifested itself in some cases as a susceptibility to Hodgkin's disease. Second, as expected for such deficiencies, bilateral descent is the significant factor. Third, certain paths are almost certainly *not* carrying the gene, despite the ancestral individuals' being members of the core genealogy, and thus, only bilateral descent via other paths is relevant. Fourth, despite beliefs in the population to the contrary, there is currently no evidence that the HD/ID cases are in any way genetically associated with those of lymphosarcoma and the other traits, nor is there evidence of any specific genetic effects in the latter group.

7.5. Linkage analysis

As discussed in the previous chapter, the most conclusive proof of a single gene is linkage to a marker locus (section 6.5). For this Newfoundland population, data on many blood-group and enzyme polymorphisms have been collected for the 1975 population. One obvious problem arises. Segregation of the HD allele among the unaffected current population cannot be detected, as the trait is recessive. Nor can a complete two-locus analysis be performed on this complex genealogy, owing to computational limitations (chapter 4). It is only among the ancestors of cases that the paths of the allele are evident, but blood types are available only for the current individuals, and not for these ancestors. In principle the solution is clear. As ancestral paths of the HD allele can be traced, so also can paths of blood-type alleles be determined, and, having inferred the ancestral paths, possible cosegregation on the ancestral genealogy can then be tested for. Statistically there may be problems; information on the ancestral paths both for marker and HD allele is probabilistic and may be unclear. In any case, the number of double heterozygotes in the core genealogy is likely to be small.

These ideas are illustrated by considering the rhesus negative allele, whose apparently positive associations with the set of 21 cases and their close relatives has previously been noted (Newton et al. 1979). For the present purposes it is sufficient to consider just three rhesus genotypes defined by two alleles, the recessive rhesus negative allele denoted r and the most common rhesus positive R_1 allele. First, the ancestry of the rhesus negative allele on the complete genealogy is analyzed, independently of the HD/ID cases. It is found that although all the information is in differing levels of relative likelihood (that is, inferences are quantitative, not qualitative), there is substantial information on ancestral paths. In particular, although there are positive likelihoods that each child of $J\&M$ may have been any of the three rhesus genotypes, there are, for some, considerable differences in these likelihoods (see table 37). Note that the three likely HD/ID carrier offspring of $J\&M$ are also the most likely to have carried rhesus negative alleles. This could be a slight indication of linkage, confirming for the ancestors an association previously observed in the current population. If the two loci are closely linked, the initial HD allele must have been accompanied by a rhesus negative one.

On the core genealogy there are two ways in which linkage with the hypothesized HD/ID gene could show itself. First, there may be segregation distortion at the linked marker locus, induced by an HD/ID segregation bias in the core genealogy consisting only of the ancestors of affected individuals. The analysis in fact includes not only the core genealogy but also segregation to the offspring of all members of the core using their separately inferred rhesus and HD/ID-type probabilities, as in section 7.3. Nonetheless, a segregation bias could remain, and it is therefore important to check first for such a bias in order to validate any apparent cosegregation of HD and rhesus alleles. For members of the core genealogy, let

$$t = P(\text{rhesus heterozygote transmits the rhesus positive allele}). \quad (41)$$

The log-likelihood for t is curve (a) of figure 45; there is clear evidence against segregation distortion, the likelihood being sharply peaked with a maximum very close to 0.5. A very slight excess transmission of rhesus negative alleles seems to have occurred, the maximum likelihood estimate of t being 0.45, but there is no evidence that this was not a chance deviation from an underlying probability $t = 0.5$.

Second, consider an association in segregation between the two loci. This could be detected via an association in the transmission of a certain

Table 37. Rhesus likelihoods for the children of *J&M* inferred from their joint descendants

Individual	Number of current descendants	HD/ID status	Likelihood		Inference
			rr	R_1R_1	
6200	671	carrier	126	62	carried r
7095	437	possible carrier	52	127	carried R_1
6606	518	—	74	29	heterozygote
7092	1,173	carrier	153	15	probably rr
7097	260	possible carrier	103	97	no information
6597	877	carrier	97	43	carried r
6267	305	—	64	103	carried R_1
6455	26	—	93	107	no information

Notes: Results are normalized to a heterozygote $(R_1 r)$ likelihood of 100. The combined likelihoods for *J&M*, normalized to a double heterozygote likelihood of 1,000, are as follows:

rr, rr	3
$rr, R_1 r$	623
$R_1 r, R_1 r$	1,000
$R_1 R_1, rr$	551
$R_1 R_1, R_1 r$	275
$R_1 R_1, R_1 R_1$	6

If rhesus and HD are linked, the initial HD allele must have been in conjunction with r.

rhesus allele and the HD allele in the double heterozygote ancestors. Therefore, for ancestors of the cases heterozygous at both HD/ID and rhesus loci, and thus for rhesus genotype $(R_1 r)$ and HD/ID genotype $a_1 a_2$, let

$$t = P(R_1 \text{ allele transmitted} \mid \text{HD/ID } a_1 \text{ allele transmitted}),$$

so

$$1 - t = P(r \text{ allele transmitted} \mid \text{ HD/ID } a_1 \text{ allele transmitted}). \quad (42)$$

Also suppose the symmetric assumption

$$t = P(r \text{ allele transmitted} \mid \text{HD/ID } a_2 \text{ allele transmitted})$$

and

$$1 - t = P(R_1 \text{ allele transmitted} \mid \text{HD/ID } a_2 \text{ allele transmitted}).$$

Again a likelihood for t is computed, using previously computed posterior probabilities of HD/ID genotypes and hence transmission probabilities thereof. The resulting log-likelihood is curve (*b*) of figure 45. If a_1 were fully in association with the rhesus negative allele (r), then t would be the recombination parameter. However, this approach can detect only

Figure 45. Log-likelihoods (*a*) for segregation bias of the rhesus negative allele within the core HD/ID genealogy, and (*b*) for association in segregation between the HD/ID a_2 allele and the rhesus negative allele. Log-likelihood differences are given relative to the parameter value $t = 0.5$; this value corresponds to no association or segregation distortion.

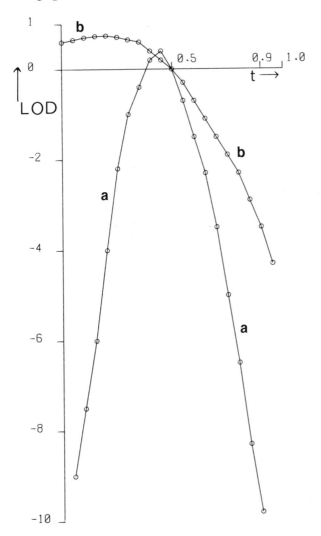

close linkage, for under loose linkage the initial association between the two alleles will be destroyed by crossovers. Nonetheless, the method provides an approximate approach to the complete solution, which would require a joint analysis of the ancestral rhesus-HD segregations. For the rhesus locus there is slight evidence of some loose association between rhesus and HD/ID loci (figure 45), the maximizing value of t being 0.2, but the log-likelihood differences are very small, and no conclusions can be drawn. Further, an association at this level is unlikely to be attributable to linkage, for crossovers resulting in an HD a_1 allele in conjuction with an R_1 rhesus allele would be likely to have occurred. It is therefore of interest to consider the contributions to the overall likelihood from the segregations in the various ancestral sibships; strong evidence for association in transmission between HD a_1 and r in some sibships but with R_1 in others would again provide evidence of linkage. In fact, all sibships provide broadly consistent evidence of no association, cumulating to the flat overall surface obtained. One small group of three sibships provides more substantial evidence for association of HD a_1 and r in transmission, and a pair of sibships shows an association with R_1. Were this evidence stronger and/or duplicated in other parts of the genealogy, it could be attributed to linkage, with one relevant ancestral crossover, but in the present case this conclusion is unjustified.

Although some of the ancestral genotype patterns are as expected under linkage between HD and rhesus, the values of the relative likelihoods are such that these phenomena are equally attributable to chance, and to the ascertainment effect of the observed association in the current population, which leads us to consider the rhesus locus. The results for this particular locus are thus negative, but they are nonetheless encouraging. There is considerable power to trace the ancestry of marker alleles on this genealogy, in probabilistic even though not absolute terms. Thus, when there *is* close linkage, it should be detectable.

7.6. Other traits: Lymphosarcoma and leukemia

Despite the above detailed genealogical analysis of the Hodgkin's disease and immunodeficiency cases, many unanswered questions remain. In particular, consider the cases of leukemia and lymphosarcoma, which are apparently not closely associated genetically with the other traits. Nonetheless, they are an "unusual" occurrence in communities of this size, and were influential in bringing the population to attention. It seems unlikely that they are an entirely independent phenomenon. Consider also the clustering of the cases in time as well as in space. For the Hodgkin's disease and immunodeficiency cases, this can be explained by recessive inheritance. Where such a trait is rare, and so only a single initial a_1 allele is present, cases will not occur for some generations. Even for first-cousin marriages among the grandchildren of the initial carrier, only 1 in 64 of their offspring will be affected. Only when large numbers of descendants marry do affected individuals occur, and the expected pattern is for cases to arise as a group some six to seven generations from the original carrier. However, in conjunction with the other traits, an external (environmental or viral) triggering factor also is suggested. In particular, the Hodgkin's disease cases could be the result of some immune-response deficiency to this factor, while the three immunodeficiency cases may be examples of a more usual phenotypic expression of the gene. These three cases alone might not have brought the population to attention without the additional "epidemic" of HD cases. All the homozygotes in the population of 1960–75 may have been affected, and it is quite likely that there were no ancestral homozygotes. But if an external factor also was significant, it is quite likely that there may now be homozygotes who will never be affected. The number of unaffected sibs of cases now reaching the adult age group is an indication of this. It may be relevant that, although there have been no recent HD/ID cases in this community, another case in the same geographical area proved to be one of the few individuals in that village who was bilaterally descended from *J&M*.

The same external factor that initiated the cases of Hodgkin's disease and immunodeficiency could have been significant in the other traits. It has been suggested that the leukemia cases, in particular, may have been the result of such a factor. One additional fact is relevant here, and may be considered either to lessen the case for partition of the traits and hence the recessive inference for HD/ID, or to strengthen the hypothesis that, while this recessive gene exists, it can have other related medical effects. Alternatively, it may be considered an a posteriori recognized coincidence. This additional fact is that one of only two unaffected members of the core genealogy who have substantial posterior probability of having been of genotype a_1a_1 was a thymoma case.

These speculations are not, however, amenable to statistical analysis—not, at least, until we gain more knowledge of the HD/ID gene. Moreover, despite convincing evidence, the aim of this chapter has not been to prove the existence of this gene. Rather, it has been to illustrate the scope and power of pedigree analysis.

7.7. Further reading

The occurrence of an unusually large number of cases of lymphoreticular malignancies in this Newfoundland population was first detailed by Buehler et al. (1975). Many details of the genealogy and demography of the population are given by the various reports of the West Coast Health Survey, and in particular the genealogical relationships of the cases are described in the report of Crumley (1977). Marshall et al. (1980) and Salmon et al. (1980) give further details and analysis, while Newton et al. (1979) report the initial rhesus blood-type findings. Preliminary statistical analysis using permutation tests (Fisher 1956) is given by Thompson (1980c). More details of the likelihood analysis are given by Thompson (1981a); the potential for linkage analysis is the subject of continuing research.

8. Sampling Theory in Pedigree Analysis

8.1. The sampling problem

In any likelihood inference there is always the paradox that the hypothesis of maximum likelihood is the one that provides probability 1 to the observed data; "what is observed had to happen" (Edwards 1972, p. 199). In most contexts this creates no problem. Likelihood inferences are made within the context of a model, which gives rise to a framework of analogous experiments that could have led to different results. Even in the case of genetic data on a single population, Mendelian segregation provides for the possibility of a different end result than the particular one observed, and different genetic models, genealogical structures, or founder genotypes assign different probabilities to the actual outcome. However, the populations studied are not a random sample, but are considered for reasons that are often related to the aspect studied. The reason a genealogy comes to attention may depend not only on the existence of the trait therein, or on there being a "surprising" number of cases, but also on the precise distribution of such cases. In this instance, one might take the view that genealogies come to attention because of their precise observed trait distribution, and hence that in order to come to attention they must show that distribution, and hence that the probability of observed data in a genealogy that has come to attention *is* one, and that nothing further can be inferred.

The whole of the Tristan da Cunhan population (chapter 5) and the Amerindian villagers (chapter 3) were studied for reasons unconnected with any particular genetic trait, but this is the exception rather than the rule. The Habbanite genealogy (chapter 6) was studied because of the observed dermatoglyphic traits, but at least dermatoglyphic *and* marker data were collected for all available individuals. The lack of segregation bias ($t = \frac{1}{2}$) indicates that individuals with the phenotype of interest were not included with greater probability than their unaffected relatives. The analysis of linkage with the marker types would not be affected even if they were (see below). On the other hand, the form of the Mennonite-Amish genealogy of chapter 4 is certainly biased by considering only the ancestry of affected individuals, as discussed in section 4.4. In the absence of information on other current individuals, a full pedigree-analysis inference of ancestral types could be highly biased. The results of any comparison of alternative genetic models for a given trait would be meaningless, for only the known recessivity and rarity of a trait justify the limitation of the genealogy considered and the method of analysis employed. The core of the Newfoundland genealogy (section 7.3) is also defined by the location of affected individuals. Although one would hope [and the work of Thomas (1984) provides some justification for the hope] that likelihood analysis on the core will provide adequate approximations to those on the whole genealogy, use of the core alone can be justified only as such an approximation. The confirmation of results by inclusion of peripheral sections of the genealogy (section 7.3) is therefore important. There is also the further problem that this population came to attention because of the number of cases involved. As noted in section 7.1, the number of cases alone conveys nothing further, and inferences can be based only upon the distribution of the cases within the population. If this precise distribution had also been a critical factor in choosing to study the population, there would be little independent evidence upon which to base inferences. In the extreme, no inferences could be made.

It is seldom necessary to pursue the argument to this extreme, but the necessity for a clear specification of trait-related reasons for considering a particular (part of a) genealogy is clear. Then either inferences can be based on those aspects of the data which are unaffected by the sampling criterion, or a correction can be made for the sampling. An example of the first approach is linkage analysis. The cosegregation of alleles at two loci can be analyzed conditionally upon the genotype at one, which alone conveys no information about linkage. Ascertainment via a phenotype of interest, and preferential inclusion of individuals heterozygous for an allele related to this phenotype, does not bias the linkage inferences. (This, of course, assumes that the model for the phenotype of interest is correctly known.) The second approach, correcting for ascertainment bias, is more complicated and requires a well-defined sampling rule for genealogies. The genealogies considered in this text represent a range of sampling criteria, although fortunately not the extreme of rigid trait-related sampling rules. For this reason, it has been possible to avoid formal consideration of sampling criteria in the analyses of them. However, the subject of pedigree analysis, and especially the medical-genetic aspects thereof, is incomplete without some analysis of the effects of sampling rules and of the choice of sampling criteria. This concluding chapter will therefore have a more theoretical flavor than earlier ones, although technicalities will be kept to a minimum. The subject of ascertainment corrections and optimal sampling is large and open-ended. The aim here is not to give an account of the standard statistical procedures that are used in this area of pedigree analysis but to explain the sort of considerations that should ideally enter into the design and analysis of practical studies. The reader will not find recipes, but will perhaps be able to take a broader view of alternative sampling procedures and of their effects upon practical results.

8.2. Sampling via probands

Suppose that a particular phenotype of a particular trait is of interest; individuals of this phenotype will be termed *affected*. If the characteristic is rare, any study of the genetic etiology of the trait which attempts to sample random members of the population will be doomed to failure. Few members will be affected, and in a large population few will be closely related. Clearly, the sampling must be via affected individuals, who may come to attention through medical records, for example. The classic sampling model of genetic epidemiology assumes that the population consists of a large number of genetically independent families (or sibships, in the simplest case), and that affected individuals come to attention (become *probands*), each with probability π. The other members of the family or sibship of a proband are then examined. Sibships with more than one proband are described as *multiply ascertained*; obviously, the information on such families is entered into the study only once. The phenotypic data on nonproband members of ascertained families provides information about the genetic parameters of the trait, but these individuals clearly cannot be considered a random sample from the population. They are members of a family containing at least one proband, and becoming a proband depends upon the genetic constitution of the family, since probands are affected individuals. Thus the aim of the study is first to derive the conditional distribution of proband numbers and of phenotypic data within families containing at least one proband. This, then, can be considered a joint likelihood for the probability π and the genetic parameters θ of the genetic model:

$$L_1(\pi, \theta) = \Pi\,[P(\text{data} \mid \pi, \theta, \text{at least one proband})], \qquad (43)$$

where the product is over the ascertained families.

In a large population approximating a collection of separate families, in studies where ascertainment is through records of affected individuals, equation (43) is an appropriate form of likelihood. The same principle can be extended to larger genealogies, to cases where the probability of an individual's becoming a proband depends upon characteristics other than his trait phenotype alone, and to situations in which ascertainment is dependent upon family structure and where family structure can itself be affected by the trait distribution within it. (As usual, references are provided at the end of the chapter). However, equation (43) provides a conditional likelihood, conditioned not only (as is necessary) upon at least one proband in observed families but also upon the collection of families which has chanced to be ascertained. Under the sampling model, the numbers, sizes, and possibly even the structures of ascertained families are random variables, whose distributions depend upon the ascertainment probability

π and upon some components of the genetic parameters θ. The distributions depend also upon the sizes and shapes of the families in the population at large; the parameters of these demographic distributions will be denoted by Δ. The probability of the numbers observed therefore provides a likelihood for all these parameters. The complete likelihood was given first by Bailey (1951) and takes the form

$$L_2(\Delta, \pi, \theta) = P(\text{number and structures of families} \mid \Delta, \pi, \theta)\, L_1(\pi, \theta). \quad (44)$$

The major practical problem with equation (44) is that new parameters are introduced. The demographic parameters Δ may be many, and their values uncertain. Therefore, the conditional likelihood [equation (43)] may be preferred; inferences based upon it will be more robust against departures from the model than inferences based upon the full likelihood [equation (44)].

Further, where there is no external information about Δ, in many examples little is lost (in terms of theoretical statistical information) by using (43) rather than (44). In large samples the estimates of parameters may scarcely differ under the two approaches, but there is an inferential difference between the two, and in general they can produce different results. Moreover, external demographic information can alter estimates. Family-size distributions among ascertained families, as compared with those in the population at large, can provide tests of the ascertainment process (Stene 1981). Clear information about population size can alter estimates of the probability of ascertaining certain numbers of families, and hence indirectly influence estimates of genetic parameters. Another approach to the nuisance parameters Δ is to integrate them out with respect to some prior distribution. There are, in fact, conditions under which this procedure leads to the usual conditional likelihood [here equation (43)]. This may be a convenient rationalization of the conditional likelihood, but it seems a little illogical to condition or integrate out the parameter Δ while considering the nuisance parameter π jointly with θ.

A more fundamental difficulty in the classical "π model" approach lies in its application to small populations such as those considered in this text. The population cannot then be considered a collection of independent families. Its genealogy is an interrelated whole, some possibly biased part of which is studied. In some cases a sequential approach to data collection is closer to reality than the classical model of random probands. It is seldom the case that total sample size is as random as the classical model dictates. Financial and statistical criteria will normally predetermine the approximate size of a study, independently of the population distribution and genetic factors involved. Even if equation (43) provides an accurate approximation to the required likelihood, its derivation as a conditional likelihood in a large population containing randomly ascertained families is unappealing. Alternative sampling models are unlikely to lead to very different genetic conclusions where a clear inference is possible, but they can provide an alternative view of the sampling process. This is necessary if alternative sampling procedures are to be compared.

8.3. Sequential sampling

Many studies arising in pedigree analysis are at least partially sequential. A group of individuals comes to attention because of a particular pattern of phenotypes. Some relatives are then studied. If data of interest are found, a decision may be made to collect further data on a large genealogy. If nothing is found, it may be considered not worthwhile to pursue the family further. It is important to assess how such a procedure biases inferences, and the perhaps surprising conclusion is that it need not do so.

Consider the following four nongenetic examples:

(a) Suppose that the probability that a given coin shows heads when tossed is an unknown number $q (0 < q < 1)$. The parameter q is to be estimated by repeated tosses of the coin. The usual experiment might be to toss the coin n times, and a result of r heads in these n tosses might be observed. On the other hand, it might be decided that the coin is to be tossed until r heads have been obtained, and the result would then be that n tosses are required. The first is a fixed-sample rule; the second is sequential, the continuation of tossing being dependent upon results to date. The likelihood, as a function of q, is the same in both cases, however. In either case, r heads and $(n - r)$ tails are observed, and the likelihood is proportional to $q^r(1 - q)^{n-r}$. The maximum likelihood estimate of q is r/n in each case. The statistical properties of the likelihood functions and estimates differ, since in the first case r is random and in the second case n is. The probability distributions are not the same, but the function resulting from a particular series of tosses is.

(b) Other sequential procedures can be used in situation (a). It may be decided that the coin is to be tossed n_1 times. If the current proportion of heads recorded is greater than 50 percent, the coin will be tossed a further n_2 times. If the proportion at that stage is greater than 50 percent, it will be tossed a further n_3 times, and so on. It is perhaps less intuitively clear that this does not alter the likelihood, but it does not. If q is large sampling may continue for some time, whereas if it is small, probably only the first n_1 tosses will be made. But whatever the sample of tosses, each has probability q of showing a head, and $(1 - q)$ of showing a tail, and different tosses give independent results. Provided all the results are included in the likelihood, the procedure that gave rise to the particular sequence of tosses is irrelevant.

(c)   Consider now a large collection of coins, all with the same unknown q value. The coins are tossed; those showing a head are tossed again; those showing a head yet again are tossed yet again; and so on. All the results of all the tosses are recorded. The experiment ceases when there are no longer any coins in play, or simply at some arbitrary point at which the experimenter becomes tired. At first glance, this procedure might appear to bias q in favor of larger values, but it does not. Every toss of every coin has probability q of showing a head. In a total set of n tosses, r of which show a head, the likelihood is again $q^r(1 - q)^{n-r}$, and the past history of particular coins is irrelevant. Provided the results of all the tosses of all the coins are included in the count, q can be validly estimated from the likelihood function (the maximum likelihood estimate again being r/n).

(d)   Suppose now that coins have a very curious property. Each starts with a probability q of showing a head when tossed, but the result of the toss affects the probability q for the next toss of the same coin. If a head is obtained, the probability increases to $(1 + q)/2$; if a tail is obtained, it decreases to $q/2$. This process continues each time the coin is tossed. The same experiment as in (c) is performed. The actual results obtained now have a different probability distribution, one that is substantially biased toward the observation of more heads, since only those coins showing heads are retossed, and these have an ever-increasing probability of doing so again. The experiment will last longer, or the point of exhaustion of the experimenter has higher probability of being reached. Nonetheless, within the context of the model, q can be validly estimated. If n_i coins are tossed for the ith time, and r_i of these show heads, the likelihood is proportional to

$$\Pi_i[q_i^{r_i}(1 - q_i)^{n_i - r_i}],$$

where $q_i = (1 + q_{i-1})/2$ and $q_1 = q$. That is, the sequential procedure leads to observation of a higher proportion of heads, but the likelihood takes account of this through the model for changing q and does not depend upon the sequential procedure per se. It still yields a valid estimate of q, provided the results of all the tosses made are included in it.

The analogy with sequential observation on a genealogy should now be clear. Observation of affected individuals alters the probabilities of phenotypes for relatives, and the aim in sequential sampling is often to observe more affected individuals. The objective of this strategy is not to bias inferences in any particular direction, but simply to provide more information about the parameters of the genetic model. For a trait caused by a rare allele, no information on penetrance or on linkage will be obtained from those parts of the genealogy where it is not segregating. Provided that

(i)   no observation is made because of prior knowledge of the result (that is, knowledge outside the context of predictions under the genetic model); and

(ii)   all observations made are included in the likelihood,

then within the context of the class of genetic models considered, the likelihood is unaltered by the sequential process. As in the coin-tossing examples described above, the likelihood is simply the probability that the observed phenotypic data will appear on the observed genealogical structure.

Criteria (*i*) and (*ii*) are easier to formulate than to implement strictly. Rule (*ii*) may even appear simplistic, but in practical contexts "data" and "observation" can vary in degree. A tendency toward certain phenotypic distributions may appear in studies that come to be published. Other genealogies may have been studied, without any but the disappointed observer being aware of the fact. Nonetheless, within the context of a single study it is clear that all results must be included in the analysis if bias is not to occur. The precise meaning of rule (*i*) is less clear, and in the case of medical traits of large phenotypic effects, less easy to ensure. The decision to observe an individual can be made on the basis of observations noted to date, and hence individuals with high probabilities of being affected can be chosen. This is analogous to the decision to retoss only the coins showing heads in example (*d*). What must *not* be done is to sample individuals or a branch of the genealogy because of prior evidence that the trait is segregating there. Practitioners are well aware of hearsay evidence such as "Uncle Fred had a son with the same problem." While Uncle Fred and his son may provide valuable evidence about the genetic model, observation of them as a result of such evidence can bias the likelihood. It would be as if, in example (*c*) or (*d*), one were told to retoss a particular coin because sudden foresight has revealed that on the next occasion it will come down heads. Only if a sampling rule is employed that leads to Uncle Fred and his son only on the basis of data on individuals already examined is no correction to the likelihood required. For example, it might already be the policy that all uncles and first cousins of affected persons will be studied where readily available, or even that all uncles called Fred will be examined. Provided the availability (and the name Fred) are not associated with the trait, no problem arises. For these pragmatic reasons, sequential sampling can be employed most easily for traits without major phenotypic effect. An ideal example is a biochemical trait for which observation is very expensive. The greater efficiency obtainable through sequential sampling will be important, and since "observation" will be impossible without a positive decision to sample, the two rules (*i*) and (*ii*) will be easy to fulfill.

The two rules do not allow for any initial ascertainment. In the case of sampling through affected probands, these individuals are sampled precisely because of their own phenotypes, in contravention to rule (i), and the likelihood must be adjusted to allow for this. For a single genealogy sampled by extension from a single initiating event and in a large population, correction of the likelihood straightforward:

P(data on genealogy | initial ascertainment)
$= P$(data on genealogy including initial event)

$$/ P(\text{initial event}), \quad (45)$$

from the definition of conditional probability (appendix 1). Provided the initial ascertainment event (the reason the genealogy came to attention) can be identified, the only correction required is the division of the likelihood by the model-dependent probability of the event. This could be simply the probability of an affected individual (for a single proband). It could be a pair of affected sibs, or an aunt-nephew pair, or any other specifiable initiating combination of similar form. However, it is important to distinguish between a single multiple event of this kind, sometimes known as *multiplex* ascertainment, and *multiple ascertainment* of a pedigree from several source events. The latter is a far more complex problem (see below).

The situation is also more complicated if the event is the knowledge that "in a large genealogy there are 23 cases," for this does not provide a specified core from which the sampling can then be extended. In some cases the correction factor may not be model dependent. For example, in linkage analysis ascertainment may be through one trait so that the recombination fraction to be estimated does not enter into the denominator of (45). Alternatively, the factor may be constant over the particular parameter combinations of interest. For example, perhaps only hypotheses providing equal population frequencies of the trait [P(affected individual)] are to be compared. In the case of ascertainment through a single affected proband, the denominator in (45) is then irrelevant to the comparison of alternative hypotheses, since it will cancel in any likelihood ratio. However, the fact that correction is in principle present should be recognized.

After the initial ascertainment, sampling (and stopping) decisions can be made sequentially. That is, they can be made on the basis of data observed to date without affecting the likelihood. It therefore becomes possible to observe individuals who are likely to be informative about hypotheses of interest, and to cease sampling when little further information is expected. Sampling may thereby be made much more efficient. Rather than address broad and impractical questions of what structures are *overall* most efficient, it seems useful to develop particular strategies for particular hypotheses and data observations.

Despite the simplicity of sequential sampling, this method does not resolve the major question of multiple ascertainment, either in principle or in practice. Where the sampling rule is such that it is possible for separately sampled pedigrees to coalesce, this probability of doing so (or *not* doing so) is part of the likelihood. Where pedigrees do not join, one may hope that the probability of doing so was negligible, returning the required correction to the single correction for the initial event. One may perhaps also hope that the probabilities are not highly dependent upon the genetic model, and hence will not severely affect comparisons of alternatives. It is, however, very difficult to justify or even investigate these hopes. Problems can arise even if only one pedigree is sampled. An individual sampled in one branch may be found to belong to another as well. This, too, is a form of multiple ascertainment, although perhaps not a serious one in the context of estimating a genetic model. Under sequential sampling, probabilities of pedigrees joining up can be highly dependent upon the demographic structure of the population, and again demographic and genetic parameters become impossible to separate. This makes usable results very difficult to obtain, and for small populations almost impossible. It is of interest that some of those who have rejected the inclusion of demographic information in the context of the classical model, using (43) rather than (44), have also rejected sequential sampling because it does *not* include it.

8.4. Measures of sampling efficiency

In order to compare alternative sampling schemes, or to decide which of several alternative observations should be made next, a measure of the information provided by an observation is required. In chapter 3 the information contents of alternative genetic systems were compared by considering their expected ability to discriminate between alternative genealogical relationships. Since the inference of relationship was to be based on the log-likelihood difference between alternative hypotheses, the expected such difference was the appropriate measure (section 3.3). More generally, for any hypothesis about a genetic or genealogical parameter θ, the value of

$$\mathbb{E}_{\theta_0}(S(\theta_1) - S(\theta_2)), \tag{46}$$

where S is the log-likelihood function (appendix 3), provides a measure of the power to discriminate between θ_1 and θ_2 when θ_0 is the true value of the parameter. Clearly this is a rather cumbersome measure, depending on three parameter values, each of which could have several components. Since, subject to certain conditions that are usually fulfilled in practice, $\mathbb{E}_{\theta_0}(S(\theta))$ is maximized with respect to θ at $\theta = \theta_0$, a convenient summary of (46) is provided by an approximation in the neighborhood of θ_0:

$$\theta_1 = \theta_0, \theta_2 = \theta_0 + d.$$

Then (46) reduces to $d'Gd$, where G is the matrix of expected second derivatives:

$$G = \mathbb{E}(- \partial^2 S(\theta) / \partial \theta_i \partial \theta_j \mid \theta = \theta_0),$$

where θ_i and θ_j are the components of θ. Here, G is the *Fisher Information Matrix* (see appendix 3), and d' denotes the transpose of the vector d, so that $d'Gd = \Sigma_i \Sigma_j d_i G_{ij} d_j$. Normalizing for the magnitude of the vector d, a measure depending on the value θ_0 and the "direction of alternatives of interest" (the direction of vector d) is obtained:

$$I(d; \theta_0) = (d'Gd) / (d'd) \qquad (d'd = \Sigma_i d_i^2). \tag{47}$$

Depending on the particular problem, one could consider the maximum of this measure over directions of d, to find what is the best potential for an observation, or the minimum, requiring a certain level of information against all alternative directions. The measure of (47) is, of course, only a local measure. In cases where the hypothesis space consists of discrete alternatives, such as for the simple genealogical relationships of section 3.3, the original form [expression (46)] may be preferred. However, even in the genealogical context, probabilities of states of gene identity by descent form a continuum, while the parameters of models can usually be considered continuous variables. Whatever measure is used, its values must depend on θ_0, the true underlying but usually unknown parameter values. The information content of a given sampling scheme does depend on the actual genetic model and parameter values; there are no universal rules. This problem is considered in the context of a particular example in the following section.

Other measures of information are appropriate to particular problems. For example, in the reconstruction of genealogies the power to exclude a parent-offspring individual was found to be important (section 3.5). Another more general class of criteria are those provided by measures of entropy; entropy formulas are closely related to those of expected log-likelihood. Entropy measures the amount of uncertainty in a distribution. On the one hand, it is intuitively unreasonable to examine individuals whose phenotypes are almost certain. More will be gained by looking at those for whom the probability distribution of the phenotypic observation has a priori high uncertainty. This is reflected in a correspondence between entropy and likelihood measures in some simple examples. However, although an observation of high uncertainty, when made, provides a high reduction in the uncertainty of that particular phenotype (by definition), it does not necessarily reduce uncertainty (provide information) about underlying parameters of genetic models.

There are, however, some variables about which low uncertainty does contribute to high precision of parameter estimates: specifically, the genotypes of individuals. Were both genotypes and phenotypes of individuals observable, estimation of parameters of segregation and penetrance would be not only much simpler but also more accurate. In section 6.6 we saw how the different classes of parameters can be confounded with each other. Unknown population frequencies of alleles obscur estimates of penetrance (figure 39), and unknown penetrances obscur estimates of linkage (figure 41). If genotypes are known, the data consist of independent multinomial observations of alleles from the population, of their segregation to offspring, and of phenotypes resulting from observable genotypes. In practice, the genotype of an individual is not observable. Thus, data on an individual contributes partial information on the alleles and their phenotypic effects, and on segregations within or to that individual. In addition, via the genetic model, the individual provides information about the genotypes of relatives whose phenotypes have already been observed, and so can clarify the information on segregations or allelic effects in previously studied individuals. Individuals who can be expected to provide a large reduction in the uncertainty of those previously observed genotypes therefore contribute more than just the phenotypic observation they provide. A criterion for sampling which considers the expected reduction in uncertainty of genotypes in the genealogy, or the genotypes of specific key individuals in that genealogical structure (the parents of a sibship, for example), is a criterion related to the efficiency of parameter estimation. The precise relationship, however, is not straightforward; even examples require more theoretical background than it is appropriate to consider here.

Whatever measure of the information provided by a genealogy or an individual within a genealogy is decided upon, it is useless without a strategy for employing it. Since that measure will presumably determine the sampling procedure, only the *expected* information can be used. Since more data will always provide more information, a payoff between the number of individuals to be sampled and the information to be expected must enter into the comparison of procedures. There may be reasons why individuals in a few large genealogies are either more or less expensive to sample than the same total number in a large number of small genealogies. There may also be reasons of robustness, outside the class of genetic models, for preferring large genealogies (giving more genetic homogeneity) or small ones (giving perhaps greater environmental homogeneity). However, as a first approximation it will often be appropriate to consider a per-individual cost, and a measure of efficiency which is the expected information on a genealogy per individual sampled. With this measure it is then possible to consider either alternative structures fixed in advance, such as "*s* sibs" compared with "(*s*-2) sibs and their two parents," or whether "unrelated nuclear families or pairs of related families" is the better option. The families sampled will of course not normally be a random sample of the population; in assessing the expected information, the distribution imposed by the method of ascertainment must be considered. Alternative ascertainment criteria can also therefore be compared—for example, single affected probands compared with affected sib pairs. Here, however, the alternative costs of implementing the ascertainment and the likely resulting sample sizes also are relevant.

Whatever the expected information yielded by a given genealogy ascertained in a given way, a particular one may not live up to expectations. The use of sequential sampling, which allows the decision to continue sampling to be based on information so far obtained on a genealogy and on expected future information, is therefore especially useful in this context. Instead of employing a fixed structure, one can consider the information that is expected from each potential observable individual at any stage of data collection. If the decision is made to continue sampling a particular genealogy, the individuals who are expected to provide the most information can be sampled, and the situation can then be reassessed. A single-step analysis will not provide a complete answer; each of a pair of individuals might be expected to provide little information, but in combination they could provide much more. The derivation of general rules is therefore difficult, but in principle much more efficient procedures can be constructed via sequential sampling. Sequential sampling also partially evades the problem that expected information depends upon unknown parameter values of the genetic model. As more precise estimates of the model are made, sampling procedures can be sequentially refined.

8.5. Applications

Using the measures of information of section 8.4, one can assess the efficiency of alternative procedures. Most of the practical studies to date have been of simple special cases, the computation involved in the evaluation of expected log-likelihoods on large genealogies being prohibitive. Whereas a likelihood provided by a single data set can be fairly readily computed (see section 4.6), the repeated evaluation required for different parameter values makes investigation of a likelihood surface substantial work (see sections 6.6, 7.3). For an expected log-likelihood, summation of weighted probabilities over all possible phenotypic patterns is required [equation (74)]. The formula also involves at least two parameter values (the hypothesized and the true underlying value), and thus many more combinations of parameter values must be considered. On fixed genealogical structures, the gain of three-generation over two-generation families for linkage analysis, or the value of a large nuclear family relative to two smaller, cousin-related families, has been considered. Other small genealogical structures have been compared for information on the inheritance of qualitative and quantitative traits. (References are given in section 8.6.) One even simpler question is that of the information to be gained from a single relative of each affected proband. Which relative is the most informative? To be specific, assume a dichotomous trait determined by genotypes at a single Mendelian autosomal locus. The data observation is simply whether or not the relative is affected as well, and the information is provided by the variation in this probability over alternative hypotheses.

Consider simple genealogical relationships whose effects are specifiable in terms of the probabilities $k = (k_2, k_1, k_0)$ of $(2, 1, 0)$ genes identical by descent at an autosomal locus (section 2.4). Let

$$Q = Q(k, \theta) = Q_2(\theta)k_2 + Q_1(\theta)k_1 + Q_0(\theta)k_0 \qquad (48)$$

denote the probability that a relative of type k of an affected proband also will be affected, under the genetic model θ. [$Q_i(\theta)$ denotes the model-dependent probability of this event, given that the relatives have i genes in common.] The log-likelihood provided by a single observation is then

$$X \log Q + (1 - X) \log (1 - Q),$$

where $X = 1$ if the relative is affected, and $X = 0$ otherwise. The matrix $\mathbf{G}$ is given then by

$$G_{ij} = (\partial Q / \partial \theta_i)(\partial Q / \partial \theta_j) / Q(1 - Q),$$

and the measure (47) reduces to

$$I(d; \theta) = (\Sigma_j d_j \partial Q / \partial \theta_j)^2 / Q(1 - Q). \qquad (49)$$

Thus, in one sense, the problem is trivial. For any given relationship k, hypothesized model θ, and direction of alternative d, equation (49) can be evaluated, and relationships providing high value will be preferred.

However, several practical difficulties are apparent. First, (49) is heavily dependent upon d. Since Q is a linear function of probabilities k_i [equation (48)], so also is $\partial Q / \partial \theta_j$, and relationships k providing a high value to the numerator in (49) vary strongly with d. Consider, for example, the simple diallelic, partial-heterozygote-penetrance model presented in table 38. Here there are two parameters (p and β) and hence two dimensions for alternative hypotheses. One way in which a particular direction of alternatives of interest can be decided upon is by fixing

$$f = p^2 + 2p(1 - p)\beta,$$

the population frequency of the trait. [Note that $Q_0(\theta) = f$.] This determines a ratio $d_p : d_\beta$ depending upon (p, β), and (49) reduces to a scalar function of p, β, and k. For unrelated individuals (49) then reduces to zero, since $Q = f$ for the relationship $k = (0, 0, 1)$. [This is intuitively clear, and follows mathematically from equation (48) and the fact that

Table 38. A simple model for a dichotomous trait determined by a single autosomal locus

Genotype	a_1a_1	a_1a_2	a_2a_2
Frequency	p^2	$2p(1 - p)$	$(1 - p)^2$
P (affected)	1	β	0
P (not affected)	0	$(1 - \beta)$	1

$Q_0 = f$.] Such unrelated individuals therefore provide no information with respect to these constant-f alternatives; on the other hand, they provide maximal information about f. Other relationships also provide zero information about alternatives of constant f; the straight line in k-space on which

$$d_p \partial Q / \partial_p + d_\beta \partial Q / \partial \beta = 0 \tag{50}$$

can lie within the triangle of k values (see figure 46).

Even if a natural direction of alternatives is specifiable, as perhaps it is in the above example, equation (49) still depends upon the genetic model θ, or, in this example, upon p and β. The values of these parameters are of course unknown. Variations of p and β (within a given f-value and over varying f-values) can substantially alter the line of zero information [expression (50)] and hence also the ordering over relationships of equation (49). For some values, unilateral relatives may be uninformative. For others, sibs may be virtually useless. On the other hand, these two possibilities represent widely different parameter combinations. The detailed dependence of (49) upon (p, β) is not so critical as the equation's dependence upon d. Within a fairly broad range of parameter values the same relationship k will be optimal.

This leads to a sequential approach. Various types of relative can be sampled (one for each proband), and as information about parameter values is obtained, the sampling rule can be refined to permit concentration upon the more efficient relationships for the currently estimated parameter values. Possible unreliability of the model will dictate that not just one type of relative be sampled, for then there would be no information with which to *test* the underlying (p, β) framework. Moreover, instead of homing in upon the "best" type of relative, the sampler would do better to focus on a few efficient types.

The above example has been discussed in some detail because it permits a full analysis and illustrates several aspects of the problem, but it is not an important practicable scheme. For rare traits, it would be foolish to sample only one relative of each proband. Presumably several would be sampled, and the decision to sample the second and/or subsequent one(s)

Figure 46. Four cases of the model described in the text, showing, in the triangle of relationships, the line given by equation (50). Individuals related to an affected proband as specified by a point on line L provide no information by which to distinguish between alternative hypotheses (p, β) corresponding to equal trait frequencies. In all cases the line L passes through U; unrelated individuals will not distinguish between such alternatives. As previously, the points P, M, and S designate the parent-offspring, monozygous-twin, and full-sib relationships, respectively. (a) The line lies within the triangle, but most relationships in the attainable space provide some information. Intermediate values of β give lines of this type. (b) Sibs provide no information; either parents or twins would provide the most information. $p^2(1 - 2\beta) + p(1 - 2\beta + 4\beta^2) - 2\beta^2 = 0$. ($c$) Case $\beta \simeq p$. Unilateral relationships ($k_2 = 0$) provide very little information, the line L passing close to such relationships. Sibs or twins would be the most useful. (d) Case $\beta \simeq \sqrt{p}$. The line L lies outside the triangle; all relatives would provide information, but twins might provide little, as M is close to L. Parents or sibs would be the most useful.

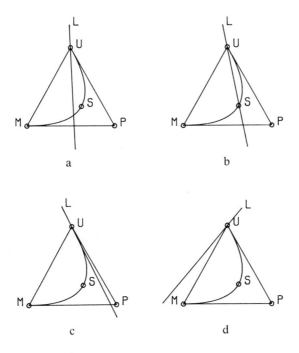

would depend upon observations made to date. Again, criteria could be developed, but again the precise decisions would depend upon alternatives of interest and on parameter values.

There are a few other examples for which explicit rules can be derived, but in almost all cases the results are not surprising. In sequential examples the important factor is normally the genotype distribution of some potential sample individual conditional upon phenotypes observed to date. Thus, in linkage examples the individuals who are expected to provide information are offspring of individuals with high probability of being doubly heterozygous. The double heterozygotes themselves are not immediately informative, but are so in conjunction with their offspring. This demonstrates one problem in trying to construct strategies in which a single extra individual is sampled at each stage. Another example is testing for the familial basis of a rare trait in an extensive genealogy. The important individual to sample is the one whose conditional genotype distribution is such that he has maximal probability of being affected under the assumed genetic model and given the data observed to date. The exact genetic model is seldom critical in determining this individual, and for an extensive genealogy without loops this criterion can lead to explicit simple rules. However, due to the theoretical and computational complexities of sampling problems in pedigree analysis and to the specific nature of genetic models and hypotheses, rules that are practicable, useful, but not obvious have yet to be found. This is, however, a potentially important research area.

8.6. Further reading

The literature on sampling and ascertainment in medical genetics is large, and the following papers provide an introduction to the different aspects of the topic. The early work on ascertainment was undertaken in the context of estimating trait and allele frequencies when sampling was via affected probands. The models of Hogben (1931), Fisher (1934), and Haldane (1938) therefore developed the subject in terms of a random sample of such individuals. Morton (1959), Elandt-Johnson (1970), and Elston (1973) generalized this earlier work to problems of estimating parameters of more complex genetic models under more complex sampling criteria, but maintained the basic concept of individual probabilities of ascertainment. Elston and Sobel (1979) extended the same considerations to larger genealogies. Stene (1981) has addressed problems in which ascertainment may depend upon the family structure rather than being a wholly individual property, and where the family structure may be affected by the distribution of the trait within it. The question of whether the full rather than the conditional likelihood should be used was first raised by Bailey (1951). Thompson and Cannings (1979) reopened the discussion as a prelude to investigating sequential sampling procedures. Ewens (1982) considered the problem in the context of the classical multinomial sampling model, and deduced that there are seldom substantial differences between the approaches; but see also Thompson and Edwards (1984).

Several authors have considered efficiencies of sampling on alternative fixed structures. Go, Elston, and Kaplan (1978) considered small nuclear family genealogies, and the important problem of robustness as well as efficiency. Moll and Sing (1979) provided a similar study for the case of a quantitative trait, and Thompson et al. (1978) considered linkage analysis. Thompson (1981b) provided a more formal analysis of log-likelihood criteria of information for the particular case of pairs of relatives.

The possibility of exploiting sequential procedures was first raised by Cannings and Thompson (1977), and was pursued by Thompson (1982) in the context of a rare gene in an extensive but simple genealogy. Thompson (1983a) placed the problem in a more general framework for the case of small pedigrees, but in the context of large pedigrees the problem remains open. However, Thomas (1984) has made a small inroad into the area with an investigation of the effects of biases in ancestral inference introduced by ignoring certain peripheral features of the data on a large and complex genealogy.

Appendix 1.
Probabilities of Events

a. Mendelian segregation

The events whose probabilities are required in this text arise from Mendelian segregation, usually at a single autosomal locus. At such a locus, an individual carries two genes, and a specified one of the two genes in a parent is passed to a specified offspring with probability 1/2. If one specified gene is passed, the other cannot be; if one is not passed, the other must be. This "choice" of gene passed is the *segregation event*. The segregation in one parent of an individual is independent of that in the other. Segregations from any parent to his distinct offspring are independent of each other. Segregations from one parent to one offspring at unlinked loci are independent.

This seemingly simple situation can lead to immensely complicated probability computations. The events of passage of specified genes from ancestors to descendants are the unions (over possible paths of descent) of intersections (over each step in a path) of the elementary segregation events. That is, the gene must be the one to be passed at *every* segregation of at least *one* of the possible paths. The passage of genes to several current individuals (and hence gene identity by descent between them) involves a simultaneous consideration of paths of descent that may have segregations in common. Gene extinction requires that a gene *not* be passed at *some* segregation in *each* path from the relevant original ancestor to the current population. Extinction of several genes is even more complex, for, were any two of the genes present in any ancestor, one or the other would *have* to be passed to each of his offspring.

This appendix therefore presents some of the basic terminology and results concerning probabilities of combinations of simple events. Although much of the text can be followed without knowledge of these results, some details of the derivations of equations require them, and they are necessary for study of some of the references cited.

b. Unions and intersections of events

The elementary events will be denoted A_i ($i = 1, \ldots, n$). The *complement* of A_i, denoted A_i^c, is the event that A_i does not occur. The *union* of events A_i is denoted

$$A_1 \cup A_2 \cup \ldots \cup A_n \text{ or more briefly } \cup_1^n A_i.$$

This union event occurs when any one of the A_i occurs; this includes the possibility that more than one may occur. The *intersection* of events A_i is denoted

$$A_1 \cap \ldots \cap A_n \text{ or, more briefly, } \cap_1^n A_i.$$

This intersection event occurs only if *all* the A_i occur.

Note that

$$(\cup_1^n A_i) = (\cap_1^n A_i^c)^c. \tag{51}$$

That is, the occurrence of at least one of the A_i is the nonoccurrence of the event that all of the A_i do not occur. Note also that the occurrence of *precisely* one (or two, or three, ...) of the events A_i is not easily considered, for $A_1 \cup A_4$ (for example) does not preclude A_2. The event that *only* A_i occurs is

$$B_i = \left(\underset{j \neq i}{\cap} A_j^c \right) \cap A_i, \tag{52}$$

and that precisely one event occurs is $\cup_1^n B_i$. For two events the situation is simpler (figure 47);

$$A_1 = (A_1 \cap A_2) \cup (A_1 \cap A_2^c)$$
$$A_1 \cup A_2 = A_2 \cup (A_1 \cap A_2^c)$$
$$= (A_1 \cap A_2^c) \cup (A_1 \cap A_2) \cup (A_1^c \cap A_2). \tag{53}$$

Intersections of elementary segregation events arise when a gene must pass through each of several segregations for the event of interest to occur. Unions arise when there are several alternative sequences of segregations, any of which would result in the event of interest.

c. Mutually exclusive events

If no two events in a set $\{B_1, B_2, \ldots, B_n\}$ can occur simultaneously, they are *mutually exclusive*. Such are the events of passage of each of the

Figure 47. Two intersecting events divided into their mutually exclusive parts

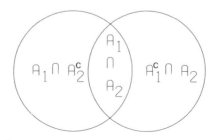

two genes in a parent to a given offspring. So also are the events of passage of alternative genes down a specified chain of ancestral segregations: if one gene is passed, no other gene can be. Thus, for genealogical genetic problems the partition of an event into mutually exclusive components is conceptually a simple task. In practice, of course, characterization and enumeration of all the mutually exclusive combinations that will result in a given event of interest is much more complicated.

If an event B cannot occur, its probability, $P(B)$, is 0. If it must occur, its probability is 1. The only other axiom of probability theory required is that if events B_i ($i = 1, \ldots, n$) are mutually exclusive,

$$P(\cup_1^n B_i) = \Sigma_1^n P(B_i). \tag{54}$$

That is, the probability of the union of a set of mutually exclusive events is the sum of the probabilities. Where events can be readily partitioned into mutually exclusive components, the combined probability can easily be found. This is the basis of Wright's method for computing the kinship coefficient (see section 2.3) and of path-counting methods in general.

Applying (54) to the mutually exclusive components in (53) yields

$$P(A_1) = P(A_1 \cap A_2) + P(A_1 \cap A_2^c)$$
$$P(A_1 \cup A_2) = P(A_1 \cap A_2^c) + P(A_2).$$

Hence

$$P(A_1 \cup A_2) = P(A_1) + P(A_2) - P(A_1 \cap A_2). \tag{55}$$

The extension of equation (55) to arbitrary numbers of events is the *principle of inclusion and exclusion*, which states that for any events A_i,

$$P(\cup_1^n A_i) = \Sigma_1^n P(A_i) - \Sigma_{S_2} P(A_{i_1} \cap A_{i_2}) + \Sigma_{S_3} P(A_{i_1} \cap A_{i_2} \cap A_{i_3})$$
$$+ \cdots + (-1)^{r-1} \Sigma_{S_r} P(A_{i_1} \cap A_{i_2} \cap \cdots \cap A_{i_r})$$
$$+ \cdots + (-1)^{n-1} P(A_1 \cap A_2 \cap \cdots \cap A_n), \tag{56}$$

where S_r ($r = 2, \ldots, n$) denotes the set of all possible subsets of size r of the n events $\{A_1, \ldots, A_n\}$. Equation (56) may be derived by repeated application of (55), partitioning $\cup_1^n A_i$ into its mutually exclusive components. In the case where the A_i themselves are mutually exclusive, $P(A_{i_1} \cap \cdots \cap A_{i_r}) = 0$ for $r > 1$, and (56) reduces to (54).

d. Independent events

The principle of inclusion and exclusion (56) is useful only if the probabilities of the intersection events $\{A_{i_1} \cap \cdots \cap A_{i_r}\}$ can be determined. One case where these intersections have easily determined probabilities is where the events A_i are *independent*. Events $\{A_1, \ldots, A_n\}$ are (by definition) *mutually independent* if for all subsets $\{A_{i_1}, \ldots, A_{i_r}\}$ for any $r \ (r = 2, \ldots, n)$

$$P(\cap_{j=1}^{r} A_{i_j}) = \Pi_{j=1}^{r} P(A_{i_j}). \tag{57}$$

In the context of pedigree analysis, the mutually exclusive events B_i are normally intersections of elementary segregation events: all distinct segregations are independent. Thus, each successive step in the passage of genes from ancestor to descendant along a given path contributes a factor $1/2$ to the probability, since a random one of the two genes in a parent is passed to the offspring. The passage of genes along paths with no common individuals also provides independent contributions to any joint event. Note that mutually exclusive events cannot be independent unless all except one have zero probability.

e. Conditional probability

Where events are not independent, conditional probabilities are often required. Examples include the probability that A_2 occurs, given that A_1 occurs; the probability that individual B_2 carries a specified ancestral gene, given that his relative B_1 does so (or perhaps given that B_1 does not); or the probability that the genes of ancestor B_3 are extinct over a specified genealogy, given that those of his spouse, B_4, are (or are not). The conditional probability of event A_2, given A_1, is

$$P(A_2 \mid A_1) = P(A_1 \cap A_2) / P(A_1). \tag{58}$$

Conditional probability is also useful when the situation can be partitioned via a set of *mutually exclusive and exhaustive events* $\{B_i; i = 1, \ldots, n\}$. That is,

$$P(B_i \cap B_j) = 0 \quad i \neq j; \quad \text{mutually exclusive}$$

$$P(\cup_1^n B_i) = \Sigma_1^n P(B_i) = 1; \quad \text{mutually exhaustive}$$
$$\text{(one of the } B_i \text{ must occur).}$$

Then any event A can be partitioned into the mutually exclusive $\{A \cap B_i; i = 1, \ldots, n\}$ and

$$P(A) = P(\cup_1^n (A \cap B_i)) = \Sigma_1^n P(A \cap B_i)$$
$$= \Sigma_1^n P(A \mid B_i) P(B_i). \tag{59}$$

That is, if the a priori probabilities of the partition events B_i are known, and the probability of event A, given each of these mutually exclusive situations, also can be found, equation (59) gives the overall probability of event A. Equation (59) is used repeatedly in section 2.6, where the events A are phenotypic occurrences, and B_i are first the possible underlying joint genotypes and second the possible states of gene identity by descent that underlie these genotypes.

f. Random variables and probability densities

To introduce the subject of random variables fully or rigorously would require a lengthy chapter. In fact, their use in this text is mainly in the context of likelihoods, to which an introduction is given in appendix 3. Here the aim is only to bridge the gap between the probabilities of simple events discussed above and the qualitative or quantitative observations upon which inferences can be based. All problems of uncountability of sample spaces, measurability, finiteness of expectations, and so on, are ignored.

A random variable takes numerical values determined by underlying chance events. An example is the number of copies, X, of a specified ancestral gene currently present in a population. The events $X = n$, for $n = 0, 1, 2, \ldots, 2N$, where N is the current number of individuals, are mutually exclusive and exhaustive, and each has a (possibly zero) probability, which can in principle be determined. The mean, or *expected*, value of X is

$$\mathbb{E}(X) = \Sigma_0^{2N} n P(X = n), \tag{60}$$

while for any function g of X

$$\mathbb{E}(g(X)) = \Sigma_0^{2N} g(n) P(X = n).$$

Hence also the variance of X can be defined;

$$\text{var}(X) = \mathbb{E}(X^2) - [\mathbb{E}(X)]^2 = \mathbb{E}([X - \mathbb{E}(X)]^2) \geq 0.$$

The expectation and variance of a random variable have the intuitive interpretation. The expectation is the value that will on average be obtained by a large number of repeated independent realizations of the same process or experiment. The variance measures the expected variability of the result around that average. The set of probabilities $\{P(X = n); n = 0, 1, \ldots, 2N\}$ determines all properties of the random variable X and is the (discrete) *density function* of X. Probability densities are denoted by f, with a subscript to denote the random variable where necessary;

$$P(X = n) = f_X(n).$$

In some cases, the random variable considered may be dependent upon alternative qualitative hypotheses or unknown quantitative parameters. For example, the number of copies of a given allele now present in a population depends upon which founder member of the population's genealogy carried the allele (assuming, for a rare trait, that there was only one). For a more common trait, the dependence will be upon the unknown frequency of the allele in the gene pool from which founder genes may be assumed to have been randomly selected. Where alternative hypotheses or parameter values are to be considered, this can be denoted explicitly by indexing the probability density by the qualitative or quantitative parameter θ;

$$P(X = n \text{ if } \theta \text{ holds}) = P_\theta(X = n) = f_X(n; \theta). \tag{61}$$

The expectation of X may be similarly indexed (the notation $\mathbb{E}_\theta(X)$ is usual) to denote the index of the probabilities used in the sum (60).

Most random variables arising in this text take discrete values: the number of copies of an allele in a small genealogy; the genotypes or qualitative phenotypes of individuals; or perhaps a more complicated function of a set of discrete genotypes (see appendix 3 and chapter 8). However, random variables taking values in a continuum also arise; for example, the quantitative phenotypes such as height mentioned in chapter 6. The discrete probabilities $P(X = n)$ must then be replaced by a density of the form

$$f_X(x; \theta) = \lim_{d \to 0}[P(x < X \le x + d) / d].$$

In the formulas for the moments of X following equation (60) the sums are replaced by integrals. In likelihood analyses, the usual focus of $f_X(x; \theta)$ is as a function of θ (see appendix 3). Whether the variable x is discrete or continuous is irrelevant.

Random variables are independent if the events that determine their values are independent. Thus X and Y are independent if and only if, for all sets of possible values $\mathbf{X}$ and $\mathbf{Y}$,

$$P(X \text{ in } \mathbf{X} \& Y \text{ in } \mathbf{Y}) = P(X \text{ in } \mathbf{X})P(Y \text{ in } \mathbf{Y}). \tag{62}$$

A necessary and sufficient condition for (62) is that the joint probability density should factorize;

$$P_\theta(X = x \& Y = y) = P_\theta(X = x)P_\theta(Y = y)$$

or

$$f_{X,Y}(x, y; \theta) = f_X(x; \theta)f_Y(y; \theta)$$

for all possible values x and y of the random variables X and Y. A consequence of (62) is

$$\mathbb{E}(g_1(X)g_2(Y)) = \mathbb{E}(g_1(X))\mathbb{E}(g_2(Y))$$

for any functions g_1 and g_2, and, in particular,

$$\mathbb{E}(XY) = \mathbb{E}(X)\mathbb{E}(Y).$$

In general, the *covariance* of X and Y is

$$\text{cov}(X, Y) = \text{IE}(XY) - \text{IE}(X)\text{IE}(Y).$$

If X and Y are independent, $\text{cov}(X, Y) = 0$, but the converse is not in general true.

g. Covariance in events

The conditional probability $P(A_1 \mid A_2)$ provides one measure of the dependence of one event (A_1) upon another (A_2). A more natural measure, symmetrical between the two events, is perhaps

$$P(A_1 \cap A_2) - P(A_1)P(A_2), \tag{63}$$

which is zero if A_1 and A_2 are independent. The value of (63) is positive if the occurrence of $A_1(A_2)$ increases the probability of $A_2(A_1)$, and negative if the conditional probability is less than the unconditioned one. Since

$$0 \leq P(A_1 \cap A_2) \leq \text{each of } [P(A_1), P(A_2)],$$

the expression (63) is always at least $-P(A_1)P(A_2)$, and cannot be larger than either $P(A_1)[1 - P(A_2)]$ or $P(A_2)[1 - P(A_1)]$.

Any event defines an *indicator random variable*

$$\left. \begin{array}{ll} X_i = 1 \text{ if } A_i \text{ occurs} & (i = 1,2) \\ \quad = 0 \text{ if } A_i^c \text{ occurs} & (A_i \text{ does not occur).} \end{array} \right\}$$

Then

$$\text{IE}(X_i) = 1 \cdot P(X_i = 1) + 0 \cdot P(X_i = 0) = P(X_i = 1) = P(A_i)$$

and

$$\text{IE}(X_1 X_2) = P(X_1 X_2 = 1) = P(X_1 = 1 \,\&\, X_2 = 1) = P(A_1 \cap A_2).$$

Thus, (63) is the covariance between the indicator variables X_1 and X_2 of A_1 and A_2. For brevity, it is often referred to as the covariance between the two events. In principle the extension to n events is immediate;

$$P(\cap_1^n A_i) = P(X_i = 1, i = 1, \ldots, n) = P(\Pi_1^n X_i = 1) = \text{IE}(\Pi_1^n X_i),$$

$$\Pi_1^n P(A_i) = \Pi_1^n P(X_i = 1) = \Pi_1^n \text{IE}(X_i),$$

and the two are equal if the $\{A_i; i = 1, \ldots, n\}$ are mutually independent events.

The type of events for which these measures of dependence arise are again those of the descent of genes, ancestry of genes, identity by descent, or gene extinction. In considering the events of descent of one gene to several individuals, covariances are positive (or possibly zero). For the descents of distinct ancestral genes they are negative (or zero), since passage of one gene at a given segregation precludes that of another. The extinction of any set of ancestral genes must also decrease the probability of extinction of any nonoverlapping set; some gene must be passed at every segregation. In this text, covariances of events are considered in the context of ancestral inference for the Tristan da Cunha population (chapter 5), and also of the descent of J's genes to the affected members of the current Newfoundland study population (chapter 7).

h. Further reading

The probability theory arising in this text is of the combinatorial kind, involving the enumeration of possibilities combining to provide an event of interest. One of the best introductions to this type of probability analysis remains the classic by Feller (1968), which does not presuppose extensive mathematical background but nonetheless goes beyond the requirements for this text.

Appendix 2.
Further Aspects of Gene Identity Probabilities

a. Proof of the inequality (16) of section 2.4

For any real numbers a and b,

$$(a - b)^2 \geq 0,$$

and hence

$$(a + b)^2 \geq 4ab, \tag{64}$$

with equality if and only if $a = b$. Equation (64) is a special case of the arithmetic-geometric mean inequality; this simple version is sufficient for the present purpose. Now, in the notation of section 2.4,

$$\psi = (2k_2 + k_1) / 4 \qquad \text{[equation (12)]}, \tag{65}$$

$$\psi = (q_{mm} + q_{ff} + q_{fm} + q_{mf}) / 4 \qquad \text{[equation (13)]}, \tag{66}$$

$$k_2 = q_{mm}q_{ff} + q_{mf}q_{fm} \qquad \text{[equation (14)]}, \tag{67}$$

and

$$k_2 + k_1 + k_0 = 1. \tag{68}$$

The k_i and ψ are coefficients between a pair of individuals B_1 and B_2, but for convenience they are not explicitly included in each expression. Further, q_{mm} is the coefficient of kinship between their two mothers, previously denoted $\psi(M_1, M_2)$, and the other cross-parental kinship coefficients have been abbreviated similarly:

$$q_{ff} = \psi(F_1, F_2); \qquad q_{fm} = \psi(F_1, M_2); \qquad q_{mf} = \psi(M_1, F_2).$$

Then

$$4k_2 = 4q_{mm}q_{ff} + 4q_{fm}q_{mf} \qquad \text{[from (67)]}$$

$$\leq (q_{mm} + q_{ff})^2 + (q_{fm} + q_{mf})^2 \qquad \text{[from (64)]},$$

with equality if and only if $q_{mm} = q_{ff}$ and $q_{fm} = q_{mf}$,

$$\leq (q_{mm} + q_{ff})^2 + (q_{fm} + q_{mf})^2 + 2(q_{mm} + q_{ff})(q_{mf} + q_{fm}),$$

with equality if and only if $q_{mm} = q_{ff} = 0$ or $q_{mf} = q_{fm} = 0$,

$$= (q_{mm} + q_{ff} + q_{fm} + q_{mf})^2$$

$$= (4\psi)^2 = k_1^2 + 4k_2k_1 + 4k_2^2 \qquad \text{[from (65) and (66)]}.$$

Rearranging this equation,

$$4k_2(1 - k_1 - k_2) \le k_1^2,$$

or

$$4k_2k_0 \le k_1^2 \qquad \text{[from (68)].} \tag{69}$$

Any genealogical relationship must lie in the region of k_i-values specified by (69); this region is shown in figure 48. As shown below, all points within this region are in principle obtainable.

b. The origin of the inequality

Although the above proof is straightforward, it has no intuitive interpretation. Why should the arithmetic-geometric mean inequality have these genetic implications? Why is there symmetry between k_0 and k_2, and why does Mendelian segregation lead to this particular restriction? A partial answer to these questions is provided by the separate detailed state probabilities of section 2.5. Seven states correspond to a pair of noninbred relatives, and when only these seven states are possible they have probabilities that are determined by the four cross-parental kinship coefficients:

state: description of genes identical (see 2.5) : probability

S_9: maternal genes and paternal genes	: $q_{mm}q_{ff}$
S_{12}: mother-father and father-mother genes:	$q_{mf}q_{fm}$
S_{10}: common maternal genes only	: $q_{mm}(1 - q_{ff})$
S_{14}: paternal genes in common only	: $q_{ff}(1 - q_{mm})$
S_{11}: maternal of first to paternal of second:	$q_{mf}(1 - q_{fm})$
S_{13}: paternal of first to maternal of second:	$q_{fm}(1 - q_{mf})$
S_{15}: no genes in common	: 1 minus the sum of other terms.

Figure 48. The attainable space of (k_2, k_1, k_0) probabilities

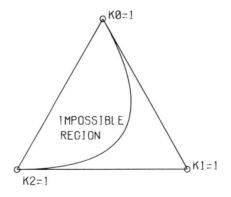

The probabilities take this simple form only because the individuals are not inbred. Thus, if the maternal genes are identical by descent, the only question is whether or not the paternal ones are also, and, due to the unrelatedness of each parent pair, the latter is an independent event. Only the four cross-parental identities are possible, and the two pairs (q_{mm}, q_{ff}) and (q_{mf}, q_{fm}) do not interact. On the other hand, genealogies can be constructed giving any combination of values (each between 0 and 1) to the four cross-parental kinship coefficients: the example of quadruple half first cousins (section 2.4) and generalizations of the same scenario provide this.

Since there are only four different probabilities, several equalities relate the state probabilities. In the space of relationships in which pairs (M_1, M_2) and (F_1, F_2) are related but $q_{fm} = q_{mf} = 0$,

$$d_{10}d_{14} = q_{mm}q_{ff}(1 - q_{mm})(1 - q_{ff}) = d_9d_{15}. \tag{70}$$

In the subspace where (M_1, F_2) and (F_1, M_2) are related but $q_{mm} = q_{ff} = 0$,

$$d_{11}d_{13} = q_{fm}q_{mf}(1 - q_{fm})(1 - q_{mf}) = d_{12}d_{15}. \tag{71}$$

Here, d_i, would denote the probability of the detailed state S_i. The two surfaces given by equations (70) and (71) are shown in figure 49. However, states S_{10} and S_{14} are genotypically equivalent: for the individuals B_1 and B_2 it is irrelevant whether their maternal genes or their paternal genes are the ones they share. Thus, in figure 49, the vertexes S_{10} and S_{14} should be "collapsed together," and similarly S_{11} and S_{13}. The result is shown in figure 50, and the origin of the parabola (69) becomes clear.

Figure 49. The space of seven possible state probabilities between two noninbred individuals

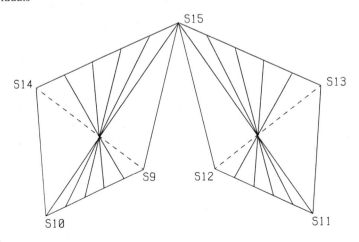

Figure 50. Reduction of the space of figure 49 combining states that differ only in the maternal/paternal origin of the genes

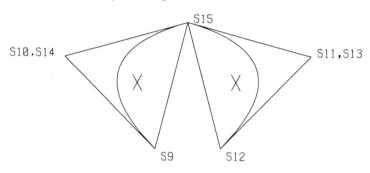

Further, states S_{10}, S_{11}, S_{13}, and S_{14} are genotypically equivalent, each corresponding to one common gene, while both S_9 and S_{12} correspond to two common genes. Combining these, the triangles are superposed, and figure 48 is obtained. Note that the same parabolic area is given by *either* of the two classes of relationship (70) and (71). Although quadruple half first cousins is a genealogically more general relationship (having q_{mm}, q_{ff}, q_{fm}, and q_{mf} all positive), its genetic effects with respect to autosomal loci are no different from those of the simpler relationships covered by (70) and (71). Here the genetic equivalence is the result of grouping the detailed identity states of section 2.5 to the coarser grouping (k_2, k_1, k_0) of section 2.4. This is a slightly different equivalence from that between uncles and grandparents, which was resolved in section 2.4 by considering linked loci. For example, a maternal uncle and a maternal grandfather of an individual both have $q_{mm} = q_{mf} = 1/4$ with respect to that individual, and are not distinguished even by the seven detailed states of gene identity by descent. Genotypically, the natural parameters of the relationship are the probabilities k_i, but genealogically they are the q_{mm} and other kinship coefficients. Whereas kinship coefficients can easily be computed on a genealogy (sections 2.3 and 4.3), direct computation of the k_i and their generalizations to more individuals are difficult. Whereas genealogies providing specified values of kinship-type (or descent) probabilities are easy to construct, the resulting state probabilities are unobvious. Restrictions on the space of probabilities of gene identity by descent (see section 2.7) are probably most easily sought via kinship coefficients, as in the example of this appendix.

Appendix 3.
Likelihood

Edwards (1972) provides a detailed account of the use of likelihood theory in scientific inference, with a special emphasis on questions arising in mathematical genetics. More mathematically oriented accounts can be found in many standard texts on statistical theory. Only an outline introduction to the ideas employed in this text is presented here.

a. The likelihood function

Suppose that relevant genetic and genealogical factors lead to probabilities of observable data, these probabilities being dependent upon parameters θ of the assumed model. Note that θ may be some complex qualitative structure, such as the genealogy itself. The data may consist of discrete events, or of quantitative values. In either case there will be a probability density for data x, denoted $f(x; \theta)$ (see appendix 1). Instead of considering this to be a set of probabilities for alternative observation values x for each fixed θ, let us consider it a function of θ for the given observed data values. As such, it is the *likelihood function*, $L(\theta)$. Relative values of $L(\theta)$ at alternative θ give the relative probabilities for the occurrence of the observed data under the alternative hypothesized values of θ. Intuitively, therefore, the values of θ best supported by the data are those for which $L(\theta)$ is large. A measure of the ability of hypothesis θ_1, compared with that of θ_2, to explain the particular observed data is provided by the ratio $L(\theta_1) / L(\theta_2)$.

b. The log-likelihood

In practice, inferences are not based upon single observations, and the data x will normally comprise independent observations over a large number of experiments. This is less the case in pedigree analysis than in many other contexts, since the individuals of a single genealogy are interdependent and it is their pattern of interdependence that is of particular interest. However, observations at different unlinked loci do provide independent "experiments." So also do separate, unconnected genealogies in the context of inferring genetic models. In this case,

$$f(x; \theta) = \Pi_1^n f(x_i; \theta),$$

where x_i $(i = 1, \ldots, n)$ are the independent component observations, which may again be vectors, and f is used as a generic expression for the relevant probability density. Hence it is computationally simpler to consider the mathematically more tractable *log-likelihood*;

$$S(\theta) = \log L(\theta) = \Sigma_1^n \log f(x_i; \theta). \tag{72}$$

This function is sometimes known as the *support function* for alternative values of θ (Edwards 1972). Normally, natural logarithms are used, as in most of this text, but in some genetic problems (linkage analysis, for example) it has become standard to use logs to base 10. Clearly, those values of θ which have (relative to others) high likelihood will also have high log-likelihood. Since for likelihoods the important criterion is the likelihood ratio, $L(\theta_1)/L(\theta_2)$, for log-likelihoods it is the differences

$$S(\theta_1) - S(\theta_2)$$

between any two alternative hypothesized values θ_1 and θ_2 of θ.

c. Maximum likelihood estimation

Since the values of θ that best support the data are those for which $L(\theta)$ [or $S(\theta)$] is large, the *best* explanation of the data is provided by that θ which maximizes $L(\theta)$, and hence also $S(\theta)$, for the given observed data, over all alternative θ's. This is the *maximum-likelihood estimate*, which may be used where a single point-estimate is required. Apart from the intuitive likelihood justification, the optimality properties of maximum-likelihood estimators are asymptotic. Under wide assumptions, where θ consists of only a fixed finite number of components, the estimate is consistent and asymptotically efficient. That is, as the number of independent observations becomes large, the estimate will with probability 1 approach the true parameter value, and will use all available information to give the most precise estimate possible. In some of the examples of this text, large numbers of independent observations are not available. Also, although the dimension of the parameter space may be finite, it can also be large. For example, in the estimation of relationships the parameters are the probabilities of all possible patterns of gene identity by descent. Thus, the practical applicability of asymptotic results may often be in doubt, but where the results are cited in the text, there are, in principle, sufficient conditions for their validity. Details of the precise conditions required must be sought in a statistics textbook.

d. The log-likelihood surface

A single estimate, albeit the hypothesis with maximum likelihood, is not normally an adequate solution. Confidence limits for estimates also are required, or a knowledge of which other hypotheses have log-likelihoods only a little less than the maximum. Where possible it is desirable to consider the shape of the log-likelihood surface as a function of θ.

The first question which arises is that of identifiability of parameters or of qualitative hypotheses. If two alternative values of θ give precisely the same probability to all possible observations, then whatever data arise, the two values will have the same likelihood. For example, in the estimation of pairwise relationships, half sibs are indistinguishable from an uncle-nephew relationship from genetic data on single-locus traits, because they provide the same value of $k = (k_2, k_1, k_0)$. *Identifiability* of k is the converse property of a problem; that is, that relationships with different k can be distinguished, given sufficient data on such loci. This is actually a nontrivial problem, considered in papers cited in chapter 3. For some autosomal loci with certain dominance patterns and certain allele frequencies, there are different k-values that necessarily have the same log-likelihood. However, since different loci have different dominance patterns and different allele frequencies, this is a theoretical rather than a practical problem.

The "ideal" shape for a log-likelihood surface is strictly concave. There is, then, a unique maximum-likelihood estimate, and the set of θ-values whose log-likelihoods differ from the maximum by less than any specified amount is a convex set (figure 51). Alternatively, there may be linear contours, and a line of maximum-likelihood estimates (figure 52). Such contours necessarily arise where there is nonidentifiability; certain different parameters always provide equal likelihood. They can also arise for particular data sets, in problems where more data could in principle distinguish the alternatives. The contours of figure 57 need not be straight, although they are whenever nonidentifiability arises in the problem of section 3.3. In yet other problems, there may be several local maximums (figure 53). In section 3.3, the log-likelihood is the sum of terms of the form

$$S(\theta) = \log\left(\Sigma_i \theta_i P_i\right),$$

where $P_i \geq 0$ and $\theta_i \geq 0$. (In fact, the θ_i's are the probabilities of possible patterns of gene identity by descent, and the P_i's are the phenotype probabilities at a given locus under that pattern of gene identity.) Since log is a concave function,

$$S(q\theta + (1 - q)\theta^*) = \log\left[q(\Sigma_i \theta_i P_i) + (1 - q)\Sigma_i \theta_i P_i\right]$$

$$\geq qS(\theta) + (1 - q)S(\theta^*) \quad (0 \leq q \leq 1). \quad (73)$$

That is, this is a case where the log-likelihood must always be concave, although not necessarily strictly so. For the genetic-model hypotheses of chapter 6 this is not the case; an example of a likelihood with local maximums is given in section 6.6. Questions of identifiability, then, are not so easily resolved.

The degree of precision that may be attached to a maximum-likelihood estimate depends upon the degree of curvature of the log-likelihood

Figure 51. A likelihood function in two parameters: (*a*) the likelihood surface; (*b*) the contours. This likelihood function is concave in the neighborhood of the maximum, and the log-likelihood is concave everywhere. Therefore, a single stationary point is the global maximum, and the sets on which the likelihood (or log-likelihood) exceeds a given value are convex.

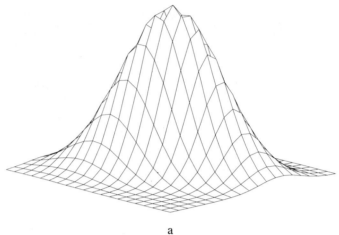

a

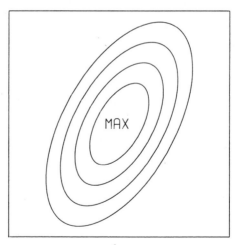

b

Figure 52. A likelihood function similar to that of figure 51, but one that has become degenerate, the value being determined by a linear combination of the two parameters. The surface (*a*) shows the "ridge" nature of the function, and the contours (*b*) are linear, with a line of maximums.

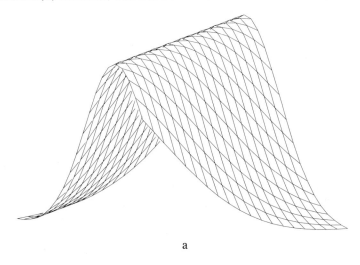

a

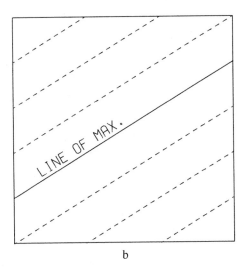

b

Figure 53. A likelihood function with two local maximums. The likelihood surface (*a*) and contours (*b*) are again shown. If a likelihood function is complex, without a detailed search of the likelihood surface it may be difficult to establish whether there are several local maximums, and which provides the global maximum likelihood estimates.

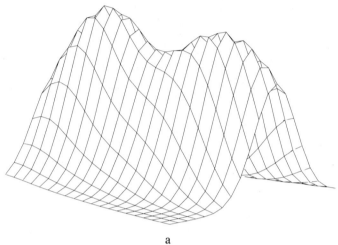

a

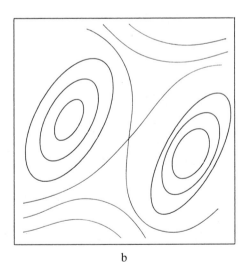

b

surface in the neighborhood of the maximum. If the surface is sharply peaked, the curvature is high, and confidence limits will be narrow. Edwards (1972) gives further details. Although hypotheses of relationship and of genetic models have quantitative parameters, it is of particular interest to compare the log-likelihoods of certain special hypotheses. For example, dominance against recessivity, no linkage against tight linkage, or half sibs ($k = (0, 1/2, 1/2)$) against full sibs ($k = (1/4, 1/2, 1/4)$). Estimates of precision are then less useful than an examination of the log-likelihood differences and a specification of those hypotheses whose log-likelihoods are close to maximal. In the case of qualitative hypotheses, of ancestral origins of genes for example, the only measure of confidence is a determination of the common features of the set of hypotheses with highest likelihoods (see section 5.3).

e. Expected log-likelihood

In considering the properties of maximum-likelihood estimators, and the degree of confidence to be placed in inferences, it may be necessary to consider not only the log-likelihood provided by the observed data but also the *expected* surface over all possible data outcomes. The expected surface is, of course, a function of the hypothesized θ-values, but it is also dependent upon the true but unknown value θ^*;

$$E(\theta; \theta^*) = \mathbb{E}_{\theta^*}(S(\theta)) = \Sigma_x f(x; \theta^*) \log f(x; \theta). \tag{74}$$

Generally, the expected log-likelihood is concave in θ for each θ^*, and strictly so, subject to the identifiability of θ. Moreover, the maximum over θ is attained at $\theta = \theta^*$, the true value. Where the expected surface is highly peaked at this maximum, a surface obtained for actual data is "expected" to be so. Thus, the shape of the expected surface provides a measure of the level of information expected from a given experiment, from a given set of loci for example.

Since $S(\theta)$ partitions additively [equation (72)] into the contributions from independent sets of data, so also does $E(\theta; \theta^*)$. Where the random variables of these separate contributions have the same probability densities, the contributions from different experiments are independently and identically distributed random variables. This provides much of the standard mathematical theory of likelihood estimation but does not obtain in many examples of pedigree analysis. Observations are sometimes made only for a single trait on a single interrelated genealogy (chapters 6 and 7). At best, observations are made on one genealogy for a variety of loci at which genes are independently inherited (chapter 3), or perhaps are made for one trait in independent families of different structure (chapter 8). In the former case, extreme caution is necessary in the application of theoretical asymptotic results of likelihood theory. In the latter, the data provide independently but not identically distributed contributions to the log-likelihood, and with some modifications and provisos the standard theory does apply. At least, levels of information to be expected from different loci (see section 3.3) or different family structures (see section 8.5) are meaningful.

Where the parameter space is a continuum, information may be best assessed by a local measure in the neighborhood of the true θ^* (as a function of this unknown θ^*). Such is the *Fisher information*, which is minus the expected second derivative of $S(\theta)$ at $\theta = \theta^*$. Asymptotically, this is also the curvature of $E(\theta; \theta^*)$ at $\theta = \theta^*$. These information measures provide assessments of the precision of a maximum-likelihood estimate (Edwards 1972). A normalized version of this measure is proposed in section 8.4. Where hypotheses of interest are discrete, the local measure is less useful, and instead certain specific expected log-likelihood differences are considered. For example, in section 3.3, $E(\theta; \theta^*)$ was tabulated for $\theta^* = k^* = (0, 1/2, 1/2)$, with two θ-values: $\theta = k = (1/16, 6/16, 9/16)$ and $(1/4, 1/2, 1/4)$. If there is a natural metric on the parameter space, these discrete measures can also be normalized to adjust for the different "distances" between alternative hypotheses of interest.

f. Entropy

The entropy of a probability density for random variable X is defined as

$$-\mathrm{IE}(\log f(X; \theta)) = -\Sigma_x f(x; \theta) \log f(x; \theta). \tag{75}$$

Similar definitions can be made for conditional probability densities. Clearly, (75) is closely related to the information measure $E(\theta; \theta^*)$, being $-E(\theta; \theta)$, but entropy does not provide a direct measure of information about parameter values. Rather, it measures the variability, or uncertainty, in a probability density. If a particular value of X has probability 1, the entropy is zero. For a discrete distribution on a finite set of points, the distribution of maximum entropy is the uniform one. The relationship of entropy to sampling strategies on genealogies is briefly mentioned in chapter 8.

g. Further reading

An introduction to likelihood theory and methodology in the context of scientific inference is provided by Edwards (1972). Many of the examples of that text are taken from mathematical genetics, and thus provide an ideal basis for an understanding of the inference approach employed in this text.

Appendix 4.
A Brief Note on Multidimensional Scaling

Multidimensional scaling (MDSCAL) is a method that provides a representation of the pattern of *distances* between a set of *objects* by suitably positioning them in a Euclidean space of few dimensions. In section 3.1 it is suggested that this method provides a useful representation of the general genealogical structure of a small population. Genealogically, the simplest overall measure of relationship between two individuals is their coefficient of kinship (section 2.3). Where there are more than about 100 individuals in the population, it is necessary to group them, and to take these groups rather than the individuals as the *objects* for MDSCAL. One natural grouping to consider is that of the sibships of the genealogy. A measure of relationship between two sibships is the average kinship coefficient between all pairs of individuals, one from each sibship. [Note that any two members of a sibship have the same coefficient of kinship with any other individual who is a descendant of neither.] A simple bounded measure of *distance* (that is, difference) between two distinct sibships is then provided by

$$(1 - 2\bar{\psi}),$$

where $\bar{\psi}$ is this averaged kinship. It is theoretically possible for this quantity to be negative, but in practice $\bar{\psi}$ is greater than $1/2$ only for the within-sibship kinship in a sibship consisting of a single inbred individual. In any case, the distance between a sibship and itself is defined as zero. Where there is no inbreeding the measure $(1 - 4\bar{\psi})$ can be used, the kinship coefficient between sibs being $1/4$, but this is usually less satisfactory, for it provides no discrimination between a sibship and a parental sibship consisting of a single individual, because that kinship coefficient also is $1/4$.

Given these pairwise distances between all sibships in the population, the MDSCAL method then determines a configuration that most closely fits them. Choice of a representation in two dimensions allows a straightforward planar diagram, and the genealogical connections can be indicated by directed lines joining the sibship of a parent to that of a child. Each sibship thus has two parental sibships, but a large sibship may have many offspring sibships, one (or more, if there are multiple marriages) for each member of the parental sibship. Figures 17 and 18 show representations of a true genealogy and of a reconstruction of the same from simulated genetic data. Estimates of the accuracy of a reconstructed genealogy, depending only upon the percentage of correctly inferred parents, can be misleading; some misassignments are more seriously in error than others. Thus, an overall close similarity of structures, as evidenced in this example, seems a more useful illustration of the adequacy of a reconstruction.

For a population larger than the example of section 3.1, a three-dimensional representation can provide greater clarity. However, such a representation is usually more successful if we consider the third dimension to be time (for example, if we characterize each sibship by its generation, or by the average date of birth of its members) rather than attempt a three-dimensional MDSCAL. The precise criteria for determining an optimal ("most closely fitting") representation of the original pairwise distances are discussed by Kruskal and Wish (1978). In their short monograph they also discuss several examples from fields other than human genetics, and many more general problems of procedure and interpretation.

References

Anderson, M. W.; Bonné-Tamir, B.; Carmelli, D.; and Thompson, E. A. 1979. Linkage analysis and the inheritance of arches in a Habbanite isolate. *Am. J. Hum. Genet.* 31:620–29.

Bonné, B.; Ashbel, S.; Modai, M.; Godber, M. J.; Mourant, A. E.; Tills, D.; and Woodhead, B. G. 1970. The Habbanite isolate. I. Genetic markers in the blood. *Human Heredity* 20:609–22.

Bailey, N. J. T. 1951. The estimation of the frequency of recessives with incomplete multiple selection. *Ann. Eugen.* 16:215–22.

Botstein, D.; White, R. L.; Skolnick, M. H.; and Davis, R. W. 1980. Construction of a genetic linkage map in man using restriction fragment length polymorphisms. *Am. J. Hum. Genet.* 32:314–31.

Buehler, S. K.; Firme, F.; Fodor, G.; Fraser, G. R.; Marshall, W. H.; and Vaze, P. 1975. Common variable immunodeficiency, Hodgkin's disease, and other malignancies in a Newfoundland family. *Lancet* 1:195–97.

Cannings, C.; Skolnick, M. H.; de Nevers, K.; and Sridharan, R. 1976. Calculation of risk factors and likelihoods for familial diseases. *Comp. Biomed. Res.* 9:393–406.

Cannings, C., and Thompson, E. A. 1977. Ascertainment in the sequential sampling of pedigrees. *Clin. Genet.* 12:208–12.

———. 1981. *Genealogical and Genetic Structure.* Cambridge: Cambridge University Press.

Cannings, C.; Thompson, E. A.; and Skolnick, M. H. 1978. Probability functions on complex pedigrees. *Adv. Appl. Prob.* 10:26–61.

———. 1979. Extension of pedigree analysis to include assortative mating and linear models. In *Genetic Analysis of Common Diseases,* ed. C. F. Sing and M. Skolnick. New York: Alan R. Liss.

———. 1980. Pedigree analysis of complex models. In *Current Developments in Anthropological Genetics,* ed. J. Mielke and M. Crawford. London: Plenum Press.

Cavalli-Sforza, L. L., and Bodmer, W. F. 1971. *The Genetics of Human Populations.* San Francisco: W. H. Freeman and Co.

Cotterman, C. W. 1940. A Calculus for Statistico-Genetics. Ph.D. thesis, Ohio State University. Published in *Genetics and Social Structure,* ed. P. A. Ballonoff. New York: Academic Press, 1974.

Crow, J. F., and Kimura, M. 1970. *An Introduction to Population Genetics Theory.* New York: Harper and Row.

Crumley, J. 1977. West Coast Health Survey. Workbook Number 2. Immunology Research Group, Memorial University of Newfoundland. Mimes.

Dempster, A. P.; Laird, N. M.; and Rubin, D. B. 1977. Maximum likelihood from incomplete data via the EM algorithm (with Discussion). *J. Roy. Statist. Soc. (B)* 39:1–38.

Donnelly, K. P. 1983. The probability that related individuals share some section of genome identical by descent. *Theor. Pop. Biol.* 23:34–63.

Edwards, A. W. F. 1967. Automatic reconstruction of genealogies from phenotypic information—AUTOKIN. *Bull. Eur. Soc. Hum. Genet.* 1:42–43.

———. 1972. *Likelihood.* Cambridge: Cambridge University Press.

Elandt-Johnson, R. C. 1970. Segregation analysis for complex modes of inheritance. *Am. J. Hum. Genet.* 22:129–44.

Elston, R. C. 1973. Ascertainment and age of onset in pedigree analysis. *Hum. Hered.* 23:105–12.

Elston, R. C., and Lange, K. 1976. The genotypic distribution of relatives of homozygotes when consanguinity is present. *Ann. Hum. Genet.* 39:493–96.

Elston, R. C., and Sobel, E. 1979. Sampling considerations in the gathering and analysis of pedigree data. *Am. J. Hum. Genet.* 31:62–69.

Elston, R. C., and Stewart, J. 1971. A general model for the genetic analysis of pedigree data. *Hum. Hered.* 21:523–42.

Elston, R. C., and Yelverton, K. S. 1975. General models for segregation analysis. *Am. J. Hum. Genet.* 27:31–45.

Ewens, W. J. 1969. *Population Genetics.* London: Methuen and Co.

———. 1982. Aspects of parameter estimation in ascertainment sampling schemes. *Am. J. Hum. Genet.* 34:853–65.

Falconer, D. S. 1981. *Introduction to Quantitative Genetics.* 2d ed. London: Longman Group.

Feller, W. 1968. *An introduction to probability and its applications,* vol. 1. 3d ed. New York: Wiley.

Fisher, R. A. 1934. The effect of methods of ascertainment upon the estimation of frequencies. *Ann. Eugen.* 6:13–25.

———. 1956. *Scientific Method and Statistical Inference.* Edinburgh: Oliver and Boyd.

Gillois, M. 1965. Relation d'identité en genetique. *Ann. Inst. Henri Poincaré* 2B:1–94.

Go, R. C. P.; Elston, R. C.; and Kaplan, E. B. 1978. Efficiency and robustness of pedigree segregation analysis. *Am. J. Hum. Genet.* 30:28–37.

Haldane, J. B. S. 1938. The estimation of the frequencies of recessive conditions in man. *Ann. Eugen.* 8:255–62.

Harris, D. L. 1964. Genotypic covariances between inbred relatives. *Genetics* 50:1319–48.

Heuch, I., and Li, F. M. F. 1972. PEDIG—A computer program for calculation of genotype probabilities using phenotypic information. *Clin. Genet.* 3:501–4.

Hilden, J. 1970. GENEX—An algebraic approach to pedigree probability calculus. *Clin. Genet.* 1:319–48.

Hogben, L. T. 1931. The genetic analysis of familial traits. I. Single gene substitutions. *J. Genet.* 25:97–112.

Jacquard, A. 1974. *The Genetic Structure of Populations.* New York: Springer-Verlag.

Karigl, G. 1981. A recursive algorithm for the calculation of identity coefficients. *Ann. Hum. Genet.* 45:299–305.

———. 1982. Genealogical Relationship: Its Measurement and Its Use in Human Genetics. Thesis, Technische Universitat Wien.

Keats, B. J. B.; Morton, N. E.; Rao, D. C.; and Williams, W. R. 1979. *A Source Book for Linkage in Man.* Baltimore: Johns Hopkins University Press.

Kidd, J. R.; Wolf, B.; Hsia, Y. E.; and Kidd, K. K. 1980. Genetics of propionic acidemia in a Mennonite-Amish kindred. *Am. J. Hum. Genet.* 32:236–45.

Kruskal, J. B., and Wish, M. 1978. *Multidimensional scaling.* University Paper Series no. 07-011. Beverly Hills: Sage Publications.

Lange, K., and Elston, R. C. 1975. Extensions to pedigree analysis: likelihood computations for simple and complex pedigrees. *Hum. Hered.* 25:95–105.

Lange, K.; Westlake, J.; and Spence, M. A. 1976. Extensions to pedigree analysis. III. Variance components by the scoring method. *Ann. Hum. Genet.* 39:485–91.

Lewis, H. E. 1963. The Tristan islanders; a medical study of isolation. *New Scientist* 20:720–22.

Li, C. C. 1976. *A First Course in Population Genetics.* Pacific Grove, Calif.: Boxwood Press.

Marshall, W. H.; Buehler, S. K.; Crumley, J.; Salmon, D.; Landre, M.-F.; and Fraser, G. R. 1980. A familial aggregate of Hodgkin's disease, common variable immunodeficiency, and other malignancy cases in Newfoundland. I. Clinical features. *Clin. Invest. Med.* 2:153–59.

Moll, P. P., and Sing, C. F. 1979. Sampling strategies for the analysis of quantitative traits. In *Genetic Analyses of Common Diseases,* ed. C. F. Sing and M. H. Skolnick, pp. 307–42. New York: Alan R. Liss.

Morton, N. E. 1959. Genetic tests under incomplete ascertainment. *Am. J. Hum. Genet.* 11:1–16.

Morton, N. E., and MacLean, C. F. 1974. Analysis of family resemblance. III. Complex segregation of quantitative traits. *Am. J. Hum. Genet.* 26:489–503.

Nadot, R., and Vayssiex, G. 1973. Apparentement et identité. Algorithme du calcul des coéfficients d'identité. *Biometrics* 29:347–59.

Neel, J. V. 1978. The population structure of an Amerindian Tribe, the Yanomama. *Ann. Rev. Genet.* 12:365–413.

Newton, R. M.; Buehler, S. K.; Crumley, J.; and Marshall, W. H. 1979. Rhesus haplotypes in familial Hodgkin's disease. *Vox. Sang.* 37:158–65.

Ott, J. 1974. Estimation of the recombination fraction in human pedigrees efficient computation of the likelihood for human linkage studies. *Am. J. Hum. Genet.* 42:98–108.

———. 1977. Counting methods (EM algorithm) in human pedigree analysis: Linkage and segregation analysis. *Ann. Hum. Genet.* 40:443–54.

Roberts, D. F. 1971. The demography of Tristan da Cunha. *Population Studies* 25:465–79.

Rostron, J. 1978. On the computation of inbreeding coefficients. *Ann. Hum. Genet.* 41:469–75.

Salmon, D.; Landre, M.-F.; Fraser, G. R.; Buehler, S. K.; Crumley, J.; and Marshall, W. H. 1980. A familial aggregate of Hodgkin's disease, common variable immunodeficiency, and other malignancy cases in Newfoundland. II. Genealogical analysis and conclusions regarding hereditary determinants. *Clin. Invest. Med.* 2:175–81.

Slatis, H. M.; Katznelson, M. B.; and Bonné-Tamir, B. 1976. The inheritance of fingerprint patterns. *Am. J. Hum. Genet.* 28:280–89.

Smith, C. A. B. 1957. Counting methods in genetical statistics. *Ann. Eugen.* 21:254–76.

———. 1968. Linkage scores and corrections in simple two- and three-generation families. *Ann. Hum. Genet.* 32:127–45.

———. 1975. A nonparametric test for linkage with a quantitative character. *Ann. Hum. Genet.* 38:451–60.

———. 1976. The use of matrices in calculating Mendelian probabilities. *Ann. Hum. Genet.* 40:37–54.

Stene, J. 1981. Probability distributions arising from the ascertainment and analysis of data on human families and other groups. In *Statistical Distributions in Scientific Work*, ed. C. Taillie et al., 6:233–64. Copenhagen: D. Reidel.

Stern, C. 1973. *Principles of Human Genetics.* 3d ed. San Francisco: W. H. Freeman and Co.

Stevens, A. 1975. An elementary computer algorithm for calculation of the coefficient of inbreeding. *Inf. Proc. Letters* 3:153–63.

Sturt, E. 1978. Rapid computer analysis of linkage data. *Ann. Hum. Genet.* 41:379–89.

Thomas, A. 1984. The use of approximation in computing ancestral likelihoods for large complex pedigrees. Knight's Prize Essay, University of Cambridge.

Thomas, A., and Thompson, E. A. 1984. Gene survival in an isolated population: the number of distinct genes on Tristan da Cunha. *Ann. Hum. Biol.* 11:101–12.

Thompson, E. A. 1974. Gene identities and multiple relationships. *Biometrics* 30:667–80.

———. 1975. The estimation of pairwise relationships. *Ann. Hum. Genet.* 39:173–88.

———. 1976a. Inference of genealogical structure. *Soc. Sci. Inform.* 15:477–526.

———. 1976b. A paradox of genealogical inference. *Adv. Appl. Prob.* 8:648–50.

———. 1976c. A restriction on the space of genetic relationships. *Ann. Hum. Genet.* 40:201–4.

———. 1976d. Peeling programs for zero-loop pedigrees. Technical Report no. 5; Department of Biophysics, University of Utah.

———. 1977. Peeling programs for pedigrees of arbitrary complexity. Technical Report no. 6, Department of Biophysics, University of Utah.

———. 1978. Ancestral Inference. II. The founders of Tristan da Cunha. *Ann. Hum. Genet.* 42:239–53.

———. 1979. Ancestral inference. III. The ancestral structure of the population of Tristan da Cunha. *Ann. Hum. Genet.* 43:167–76.

———. 1980a. Recursive routines for computations on pedigrees. Technical Report no. 17, Department of Biophysics, University of Utah.

———. 1980b. The gene identity states of a descendant. *Theor. Pop. Biol.* 18:76–93.

———. 1980c. Genetic etiology and clusters in a pedigree. *Heredity* 45:323–34.

———. 1981a. Pedigree analysis of Hodgkin's disease in a Newfoundland genealogy. *Ann. Hum. Genet.* 45:279–92.

———. 1981b. Optimal sampling for pedigree analysis: relatives of affected probands. *Am. J. Hum. Genet.* 33:968–77.

————. 1982. Optimal sampling for pedigree analysis: tracing a rare gene. *Adv. Appl. Prob.* 14:752–62.

————. 1983*a*. Optimal sampling for pedigree analysis: parameter estimation and genotypic uncertainty. *Theor. Pop. Biol.* 24:39–58.

————. 1983*b*. A recursive algorithm for inferring gene origins. *Ann. Hum. Genet.* 47:143–52.

————. 1983*c*. Gene extinction and allelic origins in complex genealogies. *Proc. Roy. Soc. (B)* 219:241–51.

Thompson, E. A., and Cannings, C. 1979. Sampling schemes and ascertainment. In *Genetic Analysis of Common Diseases,* ed. C. F. Sing and M. H. Skolnick, pp. 363–82. New York: Alan R. Liss.

Thompson, E. A., and Edwards, A. W. F. 1984. The non-equivalence of likelihood and conditional likelihood in multinomial sampling. *Am. J. Hum. Genet.* 36:229–32.

Thompson, E. A.; Cannings, C.; and Skolnick, M. H. 1978. Ancestral inference. I. The problem and the method. *Ann. Hum. Genet.* 42:98–108.

Thompson, E. A.; Kravitz, K.; Hill, J.; and Skolnick, M. H. 1978. Linkage and the power of the pedigree. In *Genetic Epidemiology* (N. E. Morton, Ed.), pp. 247–53. New York: Academic Press.

Wright, S. 1922. Coefficients of inbreeding and relationship. *Am. Nat.* 56:330–38.

————. 1969. *Evolution and the Genetics of Populations. Volume 2, The Theory of Gene Frequencies.* Chicago: University of Chicago Press.

Yasuda, N. 1968. Estimation of the inbreeding coefficient from phenotype frequencies by a method of maximum likelihood scoring. *Biometrics* 24:915–35.

Index of Notation

General Index

ABO blood-group system, 5, 38; in a Habbanite isolate, 134; in Tristan da Cunhan study population, 109–10

Age data, 21, 51, 62–63; Amerindian, 65, 66; Tristan da Cunhan, 104

Alleles, 2; assignment of, to genes, 42–43; "codominant," 69; dominant or recessive, 4; frequency of, 6, 7–8, 51; origins of, 79, 146

Amerindian study population, 47, 64, 65–69; ascertainment of, 159

Amish genealogy. *See* Mennonite-Amish genealogy

Ancestors: common, 24, 143; equivalence of sets of, 109; genes of, 77; working definition of, 21. *See also* Paths, ancestral

Approximate likelihoods. *See* Likelihood, approximate

Ascertainment: examples of, 159; initial, 165–66; multiple, 161, 166–67

Ascertainment bias, 138, 149–50, 152, 165

Association: in descent, 81, 141–43; in gene extinction, 114–15; in mating, 11–12, 48, 87; in segregation (*see* Linkage); population, 10

Assortative mating. *See* Mating, assortative

Autosomal locus, 3, 74; and distribution of trait in relatives, 4, 16; and gene survival in Tristan da Cunhan study population, 115–16. *See also* Single locus trait

Bias: in ancestry, 111; correction for, 112, 160, 166; demographic, 64; through foreknowledge, 165; genealogical, 80. *See also* Ascertainment bias

—avoidance of: in linkage analysis, 160; by sequential sampling, 164

Blood groups: Amerindian, 65; Habbanite, 132; Newfoundland, 152; rhesus, 153; use of, for genealogy estimation, 55, 66–67. *See also* ABO blood-group system; MN blood-group system; MNS blood-group system; Rhesus blood-group system

Carrier: of autosomal allele, 4, 81; of HD/ID, 145–46; obligatory, 150; probabilities of being, 152; of X-linked allele, 4. *See also* Recessive trait

Chromosomes: autosomes, 2; sex, 3, 4

Clustering, of cases, 139

Components: of genetic models, 87; of phenotype distributions, 43; in probability computation, 75. *See also* Genealogy, sections of

Computation: with assortment, 125; for complex models, 118; for continuous variates, 126; efficient, 105. *See also* Recursive computation; Sequential computation

Conditional independence: by cutsets, 91; of genealogy sections, 87, 126

Conditional probability, 13; as ancestral likelihood, 86; in ascertainment, 160, 166; for counseling and ancestral inference, 25; definitions of, 180; in genealogical computations, 84–87

Controls, matched, 140

Cosegregation, ancestral, 152–53

Counseling, genetic, 74, 150

Cousins: degree and multiplicity of, 17–18; double first, 18, 31, 53, 58; quadruple half first, 19, 33, 188

THE JOHNS HOPKINS UNIVERSITY PRESS

Pedigree Analysis in Human Genetics

This book was composed in English Times
by Action Comp Co., Inc.,
from a design by Martha Farlow.
It was printed on S. D. Warren's
50-lb. Sebago Eggshell Cream Offset paper
and bound in Holliston Roxite cloth
by The Maple Press Company, Inc.